M000210689

Speaking Up For Mom

To HospiceCare of Middletown
Volunteers
Compassion heals!
Llee

A Daughter's Quest for Compassionate Medical Care

By Llee Sivitz
and Edward Hanzelik, M.D.

Speaking Up For Mom

Copyright © 2017, Llee Sivitz and Edward Hanzelik, M.D.

ISBN 978-1-938264-17-7

Library of Congress Control Number: 2019939301

All rights reserved. No part of this document may be reproduced or transmitted in any form or by any means, electronic, mechanical, photocopying, recording, or otherwise, without written permission of the author.

One Stop Publications
6621 Britton Ave., Cincinnati, OH   45227
513-503-8965
www.OneStopPrintSolutions.com

The contents of this book are solely the opinions of the authors and are in no way intended to provide medical or legal advice, or to diagnose or treat any medical condition. It is only presented as a reference and a resource. Consult your trusted advisors regarding any specific medical or legal issues.

www.speakingupformom.com

Examining room cartoon concept by Dr. Edward Hanzelik.
Examining room cartoon, "About Llee Sivitz" drawing and title font by James Sivitz.

This book is dedicated

to Mom,

who called me her "little Lindy."

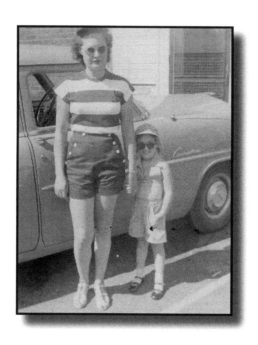

"I see a tremendous challenge when an
elderly patient enters the hospital.
No patient wants to be admitted,
of course, but sometimes it's necessary.
Yet, for an elderly person, it's a disruption
to the entire stability in their life."

- Dr. Hanzelik

CONTENTS

Preface IX

The Doctor Is In...Dr. Edward Hanzelik XI

"Mom's Story"

   Introduction 3

   Chapter One: Emergency Room 7

   Chapter Two: Doctors 9

   Chapter Three: Moving...12

   Chapter Four: Hospital 16

   Chapter Five: Rehab 21

   Chapter Six: Time to Go...24

   Chapter Seven: Moving, Again..27

   Chapter Eight: Home Caring 30

   Chapter Nine: Back Home Again 33

   Chapter Ten: 'Til the Final Day 36

   Chapter Eleven: Journey's End 41

   Epilogue 44

"The Doctor Is In"

   The Patient/Doctor Relationship

      Dr. Hanzelik On Improving the Patient Experience 51

      Dr. Hanzelik On Learning to Communicate With a Physician.....54

      Dr. Hanzelik On Treating the "Whole Patient".................57

   Treatment Vs. Trauma

      Dr. Hanzelik On the Trauma of Being Admitted to a Hospital.............65

      Dr. Hanzelik On Choosing the Best Treatment Options........70

      Dr. Hanzelik On the Crucial Role of Patient Rehabilitation 75

      Dr. Hanzelik On the Challenges of Caregiving....................78

   A Voice Not A Victim

      Dr. Hanzelik On Having a Voice in One's Medical Care............83

      Dr. Hanzelik On the Effectiveness of Advance Directives.............89

      Dr. Hanzelik On Relieving the Patient's Suffering 92

CONTENTS CONTINUED

"Nine Important Lessons"

Lesson 1 103
   Find Out What You Don't Know: A Guided Conversation

Lesson 2 105
   Make the Most a Doctor Visit: An Effective Doctor Visit | Shared Decision
   Making | What is Geriatrics? | Examining "Physician Groups" | "Personalized"
   Physician Services | Integrative Medicine, A New Alternative | Who's Heard of
   HIPAA? | HIPAA's Right to Access | HIPAA's Privacy Rule

Lesson 3 115
   Be Their Voice: What Are "Advanced Directives"? | Does Elder Law Help? |
   Is There Something Called "Patient Rights?"

Lesson 4 128
   First, Do No Harm: Prevent, Cure or Manage Disease? |
   ADRs (Adverse Drug Reactions | Aggressive vs. Non-Aggressive Care

Lesson 5 141
   Be Ready For Rehab: What is Deconditioning? | Skilled Nursing Rehab |
   Paying For Rehab

Lesson 6 153
   Consider Bringing Them Home: Medical Coverage For Home Rehabilitation

Lesson 7 157
   Choose the Right Place For Your Loved One: Long-term Care Facilities |
   There's No Place Like Home

Lesson 8 168
   Know When Enough is Enough: What Is Palliative Care and Hospice?

Lesson 9 176
   Remember, It's Not Your Journey: Caregiver Stress Syndrome |
   Parting Thoughts

"Helpful Resources"

Sample of "Living Will" 183
"DNR" Frequently Asked Questions 187
Sample of "POLST" 191
Where I Got My Information 193
Helpful Terms 197
How to Find Things In This Book 210

About the Authors

Llee Sivitz 213
It Takes a Village 214
Dr. Edward Hanzelik 215
Dr. Hanzelik On the Future of Medicine 217

Preface

As a newspaper reporter, I imagined the only stories I'd ever write would be brief - typically three hundred words or less. Yet, one snowy day in March, as I sat staring out the window of an Orthopedic Surgery ward, the beginning of an entire book spilled onto the notepad in my lap. *Speaking Up For Mom* was born.

Mom sat propped up on pillows, peering sideways at me from her hospital bed. "What are you writing?" she asked suspiciously.

I didn't dare say, "About us." So I shrugged and said, "Oh, nothing...Just notes to myself." A week later, Mom was gone.

After her passing, I put away my book notes and forgot about them for nearly three years. Then one day, as I took a walk with a friend, I recounted Mom's story. My friend was mesmerized. "You need to write this book," she said. But I wasn't so sure. Could it really help someone else? After all, don't we all go through the same things? Perhaps that was the very point my friend was making.

Looking back, I realize how ill equipped I was to handle Mom's medical crisis. My only experience with our health care system had been a brief stint as a nurse's aide some forty years prior. And even though that is more experience than most people have, I felt at sea and unsupported throughout Mom's entire healthcare journey. Yet, I saw and heard of patients (or their family members) who had a medical background and these patients seemed to have a much more positive experience in the medical setting than we did. I found this both odd and disturbing. What happens to those of us who don't know what questions to ask or what our rights are as a patient or advocate, or where to turn for second opinions or alternative therapies? Maybe you are in a similar situation with your loved one now or have that ahead of you. Or perhaps you have already travelled down that road, and along with some precious memories, you have some lingering guilt about how things unfolded. I know I did.

I originally wrote this book as a guide for my husband and our adult children, should they ever need to advocate for me. Admittedly, being responsible for another's health care decisions can be a scary thing. It is also an incredible privilege when someone trusts you enough to place their life in your hands. Yet, with so many options for medical treatment available today, it's imperative to know what your loved one wants and to recognize that as a patient, they have the right and the power to choose. We must give them a voice.

In the first part of *Speaking Up For Mom*, you can follow along as I go through a steep learning curve trying to protect my loved one in our medical care system today. I recount

Mom's medical odyssey in eleven telling episodes, which comprise the core of "Mom's Story." Next, we visit with Internal Medicine Physician Edward Hanzelik in "The Doctor Is In." Dr. Hanzelik draws upon his decades of wholistic care and patient advocacy to share a compassionate and candid perspective on giving patients a voice. Unfortunately, I did not know Dr. Hanzelik when Mom was alive. Fortunately, he is here for you.

Our office visit with Dr. Hanzelik is followed by "Nine Important Lessons." These simple lessons explore in more detail the topics discussed in Dr. Hanzelik's and my narratives. Not all of these will be applicable to you now but they may help you prepare for the future. The links and footnotes in each lesson are a great place to delve further into each topic, or act as a jumping off point for more research and learning. The fourth section, "Helpful Resources," is a compilation of information to have at your finger tips - resources that support our "Nine Important Lessons."

In summary, *Speaking Up For Mom* may guide you to a better patient experience in two ways. One, it can help inform you of what's possible for your loved one and what your role is in protecting their wishes. And two, it can help clarify and convey your health care preferences to *your* health care proxy - so that if or when that person is needed, they can be at their best for you. However, it's important to remember that just as parents cannot guarantee their children a perfect childhood, no one can guarantee a perfect outcome to someone's medical crisis or a perfect end to their days. That's just the way it is. Yet, being as prepared as we can be will certainly help.

One final thought...many people working in the medical care field, whether they be doctors, nurses, technicians or assistants of various kinds, want to make a difference. They are passionate about relieving human suffering and their efforts are often heroic. Without them, many of us would not be here today. But I now understand that every patient needs someone in their corner. The question is, are we willing to be that person? Can we overcome our fear of the white coats? Are we willing to *speak up*?

Sincerely,

Llee

The Doctor Is In...Dr. Edward Hanzelik

In *Speaking Up For Mom*, Llee honestly and openly shares her experiences of helping with her mom's health care needs and the intense drama that unfolds in the last three months of her mother's life. A daughter's role in this came to her as a complete surprise, as it often does, and she describes herself as feeling "clueless" when it came to navigating the challenges posed by the medical care system - which was the only place she could turn to in that moment of great uncertainty about her mother's survival.

As a doctor, I first started taking care of patients in medical school over forty years ago. I have seen many people in very similar situations. In fact, any one of us could find ourselves in a similar predicament at any moment, with no warning. Someone we love and care about can suddenly be struck with a major change in their health - and you or I may be the only person in a position to help with the critical decisions that will decide whether this dear person lives or not or with how much disability. I know this is a scary thought that most people do not even want to verbalize. But it can and does happen.

Usually, it is unexpected. As we get older - in our 70's, 80's and 90's - we are less robust and more susceptible to a surprise threat to our health. It could be an accident, chest pain, heart attack, high fever, infection, seizure, sudden shortness of breath, a system not working like speech, or the use of an arm or a leg.

Speaking Up For Mom describes very poignantly what it was like for Llee to suddenly be thrust into a situation where she was the spokesperson for her mother. She was left with doubts, questions, regrets and a strong feeling that it could have gone better. She is writing this book to help others, like you, see what she experienced so you can be more prepared than she was.

I agree that there is quite a bit more that we can do to have better results from the medical system. I feel the most important factor in the outcome of care is the clarity and strength of the caregivers and the people making the medical decisions to do what's best for the patient. But the medical environment is quite intimidating and the decision makers need support and even training to handle their responsibilities effectively.

I have been asked to contribute to *Speaking Up For Mom* and I consider it an honor to do so. As the author tells her story, I will convey my perspective as a doctor and I will look at what could have been different. How could this experience have been more satisfying and less painful? My hope is that you will discover options that you have if you ever find yourself in a similar situation ("God forbid," as people say, when considering such a possibility.)

I know it is possible to feel at peace, to feel clear that you have done everything possible as a patient representative and to be gratified that you were able to make the best decisions for your loved one. My hope is that my commentary will help instill that confidence in you.

With kind regards,

Dr. Hanzelik

"Mom's

Story"

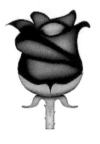

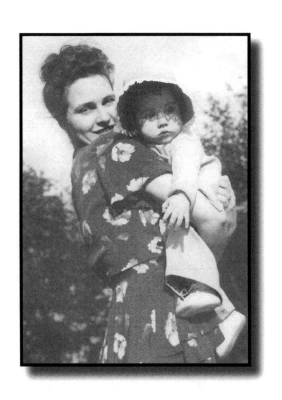

Introduction

Mom was deathly afraid of doctors, and perhaps she had good reason to be. When she was just thirty-five years old and I was nine, her health took a downward turn. She lost considerable weight and seemed to have no energy to make it through the day. Eventually, Dad took her to a doctor and the doctor gave her allergy shots for almost a year. Then she started coughing up blood. So Dad took her to a second doctor who recognized right away that Mom had an advanced case of tuberculosis. In an eerie twist of fate, Mom's own mother had died of the disease when Mom was my age, and Mom had subsequently been raised by a foster family. So I can only imagine what was going through her mind when she heard this second doctor's diagnosis.

Fortunately, medicine had progressed by the time Mom fell ill, and radical surgery - removing her left lung - saved her life. Unfortunately, however, the health policy of the day dictated that she be quarantined for two years in a sanitarium that was eighty miles from our house. So every Sunday, Dad and I made the two-hour drive out to the countryside to see her, and since I was too young to be allowed inside the sanitarium, I'd stand in the building's parking lot and wave to her as she looked down from her sixth floor window. I saw Mom cry a lot, but perhaps it was as much about realizing how sad her own mother felt leaving her, as it was about missing me. At any rate, when Mom was finally allowed to come home, she never spoke of her illness again - and she never went to another doctor.

As an only child, especially during my early years before Mom got sick, she and I were practicably inseparable. We were often left at home all day because Dad took the family car to work. So in the morning, I would watch Mom wind her hair into tight little pin curls, cover them carefully with a scarf and then spent all day washing, ironing and cleaning. In the evening, she would style her hair, put on a dress and high heels and greet Dad at the door. It was sort of like living in a 1950's tv sitcom, but without any of the jokes or laugh tracks. Mom tried hard to be the perfect housewife, yet I could tell that she wanted more out of life - independence, new experiences and freedom. So her relationship with Dad was pretty strained because, well, he wanted to be the boss.

Regrettably, once Mom returned home from the sanitarium, the relationship between she and I became strained as well. I was no longer the little girl she had left behind, and I felt self-conscious and awkward around her. As my hormones raged into puberty, she seemed out of touch with my world, and like many girls of my generation, I was determined to break the 1950's housewife mold. I often criticized her for not standing up to Dad and for not "getting a life". And sadly, more than once, my tirades brought her to tears.

However, despite all the family turmoil, something inside Mom must have stirred. When

I left for college, she took a temporary job wrapping Christmas packages at our local post office. This led to full-time employment and later a burgeoning career as Administrative Assistant to the Postmaster. She oversaw hiring of all his employees, had a personal secretary and managed an impressive operating budget. But more importantly, her self-esteem soared. She invested in a new wardrobe, kept a weekly salon appointment, drove her own car, opened her own bank account and made new friends. In fact, she often said that that job was her "freedom" and I think one of her greatest regrets was having to leave it all behind to retire to Florida with Dad.

In the meantime, after college, I didn't return home, partly to avoid the family drama. I travelled and lived in several cities before eventually meeting my husband and settling down in Ohio to raise a family. I kept in touch with Mom and Dad only sporadically, visiting them with our two young sons just on rare occasions. I think Mom would have liked to have seen us more, but she had her hands full taking care of Dad and making sure things were peaceful at home - and our presence just added more stress. However, she never complained, and it wasn't until Dad died unexpectedly a decade after they moved to Florida that I started keeping closer tabs on her.

When I did, one thing became quickly apparent. Now that Mom was a widow, she seemed giddy with her new found freedom. She purchased a waterfront condominium and decorated it to her liking. And no longer tied down to a husband who was afraid of flying, she packed her bags and took off to see the world. She visited ports of call in the Greek islands; saw her favorite singer Wayne Newton in Las Vegas; sailed on a cruise ship through the Panama Canal; and kissed the Blarney Stone in Ireland. She even rode a helicopter into the mouth of a Hawaiian volcano! At one point, she flirted with the idea of getting her own real estate license, and briefly dabbled in taking up golf. To top it off, at age seventy-five, she fell in love and eventually had a live-in boyfriend. And in the midst of all this, she off-handedly told me one day that if anything ever happened to her, there was an old coffee can under the kitchen sink in her apartment that contained her final instructions.

A decade later, the boyfriend also had passed away and Mom was alone once again and in her eighties. In contrast to the years after Dad's passing, however, this time she seemed subdued and almost reticent, content to stay at home rather than seek out new experiences. Yet, she still appeared to be healthy and thriving. And one thing didn't change. She was adamant about not going to a doctor. She swore by her few "health routines": drinking a cup of instant coffee in the morning; taking a daily baby aspirin; eating a banana for potassium; and using Benadryl for pain or when she couldn't sleep. And by all accounts, this routine seemed to be working.

I, meanwhile, was busy with a budding writing career and helping my sons through college. It never occurred to me that something might be medically wrong with Mom, or that my occasional long distance visits might not be enough. Perhaps this was due to lack of experience on my part in dealing with an elderly parent (after all, Mom had taken care of Dad until the very end.) Or was I in denial? Maybe a little of both. Whatever the reason, when at age eighty-two, Mom finally had another serious health scare, it jolted me back to reality. I now understood that she needed me.

My next five years of caregiving for Mom were filled with some of our most joyful moments together, as you will read. And yet, they were also fraught with doctors' appointments, medical procedures, and eventually hospitalizations and surgeries - everything she never wanted. Like Mom, I subscribed to alternative ways of healing, so traditional health care was unchartered territory for me. And, regrettably, she and I had never discussed what would happen if a situation arose where she needed it. Consequently, when she did, especially in the last few months of her life as her health declined rapidly, I was clueless about how to proceed. I was functioning in what Dr. Hanzelik calls "a crisis orientation" and I made some critical mistakes. Perhaps the most egregious of these was not listening to her when she finally tried to tell me what she wanted in her final days.

Ultimately, I realized how fortunate I was to take that medical journey with Mom. Despite its heartache, I gained a new understanding of the love in our relationship and a deep appreciation for how strong she really was. It reminded me of this:

As a child, I expected my parents to be perfect.
As an adolescent, I saw them as severely flawed.
As an adult, their aging was a dogged reminder of my own mortality.
But with their passing, I recognized that they were simply like me, trying to
understand what life is about.

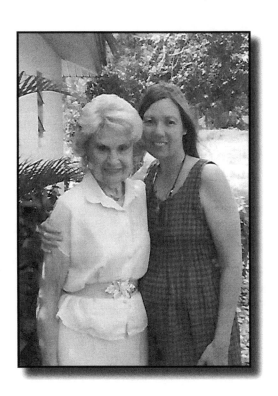

Chapter One: Emergency Room

(When things seem ok, sometimes they're not.)

As Mom entered her eighties, the most striking thing about her was her appearance. For her age, she still looked immaculately "put-together" - often wearing pastel pants and a matching top, decorative belt, costume jewelry and two large diamond wedding rings. She also wouldn't dare to be seen without makeup, and at odd moments you could catch her whipping a lipstick out of her purse and reapplying it. Moreover, once she reached age fifty, I never saw her without a wig until the final months before she died. And on all occasions, Mom's shoe of choice was heels, no matter how low they had to be (as evidenced by the sneakers I gave her one Christmas that lay untouched and unworn in her clothes closet.)

In stature, Mom was medium height and slightly built. Remarkably, she could climb a set of stairs with the best of us (most likely due to some residual stamina from her high school softball and basketball days, as she rarely exercised.) And thanks to her Alabama upbringing, she had a slight Southern drawl which Dad chided her to suppress soon after they met. She also was extremely agreeable to the point of appearing to have no opinion at all. I suppose life's situations had taught her that it simply wasn't worth the trouble to speak her mind. As a result, she got along well with everyone and people loved her.

Another thing that stood out about Mom was her uncanny ability to steer conversations away from herself. She was extremely private about her affairs - medical, financial or otherwise - and she never confided in anyone, not even me, except on a "need-to-know" basis. Therefore, as a child, I obeyed her unspoken rule to never ask uncomfortable questions - and it wasn't until much later, perhaps too late, that I realized this was her ineffectual way of coping with the traumatic events in her life.

Thus, when I visited Mom in Florida during the Spring of her eighty-second year and saw that she had a bandaid on her cheek, it was no surprise that she deflected my question when I asked why it was there. Yet, every time we went to the grocery store she made a bee-line for the bandaid aisle. I finally expressed my concern and she assured me that there was nothing to worry about. It was getting better, she said. But I knew that "it" wasn't, because each time I paid her a visit, the bandaid was bigger.

One day, as Mom and I were playing miniature golf in the muggy Florida weather, the bandaid fell off. It exposed a fleshy, ugly, mushroom-like growth about the size of a quarter on her cheek. I was aghast. She said she had been putting anti-fungal cream on it and it seemed to be shrinking. I told her it was obviously not shrinking and we needed to see a doctor but, of course, she adamantly refused. I felt perplexed. What was she afraid of? And if she didn't go to a doctor, what would happen to her?

That evening, as we sat on her apartment balcony watching the sunset, I took a deep breath and decided to broach the subject again, this time with a little tough love. "Mom," I said, "Either we get this thing on your cheek taken care of or I'm afraid you might die." Silence. As she stared at the sinking sun, her profile was stoic and unmoving. Several minutes passed and soon I could hardly see her in the deepening dusk. Did she even hear me, I wondered? Is it possible she thinks she has a choice?

After what seemed like an eternity, she finally said, "I will go to the emergency room, but I will NOT go to a doctor." Sigh. I recognized this stubborn streak at once. Yep, she was digging in her heels. It was either go to the emergency room or nothing. So the next day, we went.

Of course, the emergency room staff at the hospital thought we were crazy. The triage nurse insisted that they didn't have an "emergency" dermatologist. I responded that I knew that, but we didn't have a choice. So eventually a doctor was summoned and he confirmed that Mom had basal cell skin cancer. He said that we needed to find a dermatologist right away for outpatient surgery.

Then the nurse read me the "riot act" for "not taking care of your mother." Mom just sat there and didn't say a word.

Chapter Two: Doctors

(Present fears are often rooted in the past.)

It had been a week since we heard the emergency room edict that Mom needed to find a dermatologist for out-patient surgery on her cheek. However, she refused to go to a woman doctor or to a physician with a foreign sounding name. So we combed the city looking for the appropriate male physician who would also accept new patients (which in Florida, with its high incidence of skin cancer, was like finding a needle in a haystack.) At one point, I got so desperate, I called my husband in Ohio and he searched the internet until he found a doctor who fit the bill. Relieved, I was able to schedule Mom's out-patient surgery right away.

The night before the surgery, as I was getting ready for bed, there was a knock on my bedroom door. I opened it to find Mom standing there - barefoot and in her nightgown - looking very forlorn.

"Do I have to go?" she pleaded.

"Yes," I said, as firmly as I could. This was a defining moment. For the first time in my life, I felt uncomfortably like Mom's parent rather than her child. As I watched her obediently pad back to bed, I shook my head. Obviously, she dreaded going to the doctor, but why? It didn't occur to me that perhaps her fear was not so much about her current situation as it was about her past.

I wasn't allowed to be with Mom during the skin surgery, but she acted brave and the doctor said she did fine. I figured that she must have been at least a tiny bit relieved to have that awful thing off her cheek! For the next month, she took her preventative antibiotics and followed the rather complicated wound care instructions as best she could. When the time came for her follow-up appointment, however, she asked me to come along - so I flew down to Florida again.

One night, before the appointment, we were out to dinner and Mom said she wanted to show me something. She pointed to a spot on her leg that looked a lot like the cancerous growth that had been on her cheek. And she said it was growing fast. Truthfully, I wasn't surprised by this. Raised in the South, Mom had always been a sun worshiper. And as far back as I could remember, she sunbathed each summer until she sported a dark, golden tan. When she moved to Florida with Dad, she found herself in the land of perpetual summer and she loved it. Unfortunately, those years of tanning and skin damage had finally caught up with her.

So I delayed my flight home and we scheduled out-patient surgery for the tumor on her leg. Mom went through another operation and, after I left, another month-long stint of wound care and antibiotics. When it came time for the follow-up appointment, I suggested that she could go without me. She retorted that it was too far to drive, the taxis charged her outrageous fares, and the city busses were unsafe. I mentioned Senior Services as a possibility, but she vehemently declared that this would embarrass her in front of her neighbors. So I flew down to Florida again. At this follow-up appointment, the doctor discovered *seven* more basal cell tumors. I was grateful that Mom no longer balked at the prospect of getting them removed. Yet, I saw clearly that my involvement was key to her cooperation. So I reluctantly put my writing career and my family in Ohio on hold to focus on her recovery. Over the next two years, I spent twelve extended stays in Florida coaxing her through several surgeries and the follow up appointments that went with them.

Amid all these medical procedures and doctor visits, however, Mom and I had some very memorable times. It was almost like my childhood days all over again, when we had been inseparable. We went to the movies and saw "Dream Girls" and "Walk the Line". We dined at Denny's so she could get the "Senior Special". We coupon-shopped at Walgreen's for Kleenex and aspirin. And we had pizza delivered and ate it while watching "Wheel of Fortune." Sometimes, we took walks in the park and held hands. Sometimes, we got the giggles over silly things and laughed till we cried. And we hardly ever missed a sunset.

Once the surgeries were over, the dermatologist told Mom that she needed to get a physical exam. Mom didn't think so. And I agreed with her. She hadn't seen a family doctor in years and she seemed fine except for the skin cancers. But I began to second-guess myself (was that emergency room nurse still haunting me?) and I eventually suggested to Mom that maybe we should follow the doctor's advice. This was, unfortunately, the beginning of a very regrettable pattern - going against my gut feelings, and more importantly, ignoring hers, to comply with a physician's wishes.

We decided to go to a health clinic near Mom's condo, on the outside chance that she might be able to drive to her future appointments. As it turned out, a clinic wasn't the best choice because each time she went there, she was seen by a different physician, so none of them really got to know her. On the first visit, Mom had a psychological evaluation. The doctor asked her where she lived and who the President was. Mom was her usual charming self and passed the test with flying colors. I was somewhat surprised at this because, since undergoing her skin surgeries, Mom's behavior had begun to change. Sometimes while we were watching TV, she'd ask me the same thing over and over. And she insisted on having the newspaper delivered, although I knew she wasn't reading it any more. And why was she up at two in the morning, checking the lock on the front door? These things perplexed me but unfortunately I didn't dare mention them to her or to her doctor. And neither did she.

The doctor prescribed low doses of four different daily medications and told me not to worry about Mom's heart arrhythmia. What?? I didn't even know Mom had a heart arrhythmia!! (I can now appreciate that these Florida physicians seemed a little more experienced than their northern counterparts when it came to prescribing, or not prescribing, certain drugs and procedures for elderly patients.)

Then the doctor ordered an ultrasound of Mom's heart. She laid down on a cot, and the tech came in and moved a metal wand over her chest while he stared at the ultrasound screen. After a while, he told her to roll over on her side. Then he told her to roll onto her other side. I could tell Mom was getting perturbed, so I asked if there was a problem.

"I can't find her heart," he said.

"Is that a problem?" I asked, and the three of us burst out laughing. With that, the tech left the room and came back with his supervisor. The supervisor read Mom's chart and then moved the wand down to her waist. Sure enough, there was her heart! Because Mom's left lung had been removed during her tuberculosis surgery many years before, there was nothing to hold her heart up.

When we came out of the exam room, the clinic staff was gathered around Mom's ultrasound picture and the doctor was waving his hand at it and explaining with aplomb that this was the way doctors used to treat tuberculosis in the 1950's, before there was medication. I could feel Mom dying of embarrassment. It never ceased to amaze me how doctors could talk about Mom right in front of her as if she wasn't there.

Chapter Three: Moving

(Change requires understanding.)

Mom's visit to the emergency room about her skin cancer led to nine out-patient surgeries over a two-year period. Her subsequent routine physical exam by a primary care physician had resulted in multiple prescriptions for hypertension and cholesterol, and numerous follow-up doctor visits.

Now, at the age of eighty-four, Mom seemed different. It was almost as if she had experienced some kind of trauma in the last two years that had accelerated her decline, although I didn't know what it was. Her memory problems appeared to be getting worse and the only thing she seemed to care about, which she mentioned with increasing regularity, was that she "loved her condo." This comment was so pointed, I was certain that she was trying to tell me something, but it was as if she was speaking in a secret code and I was clueless as to what it meant.

Several weeks after Mom's last skin surgery, I flew down to Florida to see how she was doing. To my dismay, I discovered that she had stopped driving - and had apparently run out of food. Mom often declared to me that driving was her ticket to freedom and she would never give it up. Yet, I had no idea how good of a driver she was, since she always insisted that I be the driver when I was in town. So this new development perplexed me. Did she get lost on her way to the grocery store? Or have a near miss with another car? Did she forget how to park or how to fill up the gas tank? To this day, I don't know what caused her to stop driving because she never told me.

Whatever the reason, this not-driving thing was a big deal. As I mentioned before, public transportation was not an option with Mom and she shuddered at the thought of her neighbors seeing Meals on Wheels at her door. Once, when I brought up the topic of long-term care, she glared at me as if I was sending her to the firing squad. So I was pretty sure that she hadn't any plans for this new juncture in her life, except (ah…now I understood) she "loved her condo."

In light of this new situation, I begged her to let me research some local senior services and/or retirement communities. Looking back, I think she said yes to this only to pacify me and stall for time, as she really had no intention of agreeing to any of it. Having previously visited friends in assisted living facilities, she had already crossed that option off her list. Perhaps those places reminded her too much of her past experience in the sanitarium.

At any rate, with my hopes up, I flew back to Ohio and optimistically returned to Florida a few days later with a list of places to check out. I hardly made it through the door before Mom told me that she was glad to see me BUT she wasn't going to visit any "old age homes." And she didn't want any senior services either. In fact, she didn't want to change a thing. And, by the way, she loved her condo.

Flummoxed, I stocked up her kitchen with as many groceries as it would hold, paid her a short visit and dejectedly flew home.

Two days later, Mom called me. She said she hadn't felt "so blue" in a long time and she didn't know why...she just felt really down. I tried to console her, but I also knew I couldn't continue to travel to Florida every two weeks to buy her groceries. So I said I'd call back once I thought of something. My husband suggested that perhaps she could move to Ohio and live with us. (Where did I find someone like this, right?) It was such a sweet offer, and yet every fiber of my being resisted. After two years of long-distance care, I was emotionally and physically drained and I didn't know if I could continue with caregiving on a weekly, and possibly daily, basis. However, since Mom was refusing outside help and I was her only child and the only family she had, what else could I do?

So I called back and told her that I thought she had two choices - either to move up north with us or starve to death. I know that sounds unkind, but I tried to say it in a nice way, and not betray the fact that I was fighting my own urge for survival to even suggest it. Perhaps she sensed my desperation, because she stated emphatically that she would NOT move - and then she hung up on me. I admit, I felt almost relieved. Yet, I knew something had to give. So my husband mailed her a handwritten note saying how much we wanted her to be with us as a part of our family (I know, again, amazing, right?) and it worked. After a few days, she called back and said she looked forward to coming. But she insisted on having her own place. She would not live with us.

Luckily, there was a condominium apartment available for rent just a mile from our house. It was on the twelfth floor and had a lovely view. However, it needed a lot of work. So we rented it, and for the next week I cleaned and painted the entire place and moved in a few pieces of furniture. Then it was time to pick up Mom.

My husband agreed to help me, so the next day I flew down to Florida ahead of him to get Mom ready. When I got there, you guessed it, she told me that she had changed her mind and she wasn't going anywhere. It was all I could do to keep my composure as I explained that she couldn't stay in Florida by herself. So she finally gave in, but she made it clear that she wasn't happy about it and she wasn't going to help us with the move.

Looking back, I had no idea what she was giving up by moving from her home in Florida to a place in wintry Ohio that she had never seen, or what a step down this would be in her independence. My declaration alone that she could no longer live in Florida by herself must have been a huge blow to her ego. Could she have made other choices that would have made it easier for her to stay where she was? Perhaps so, but those were choices she was not willing to make.

The next day my husband arrived and we started packing up Mom's belongings. True to her word, she hid in her bedroom and made herself scarce during the entire process (which didn't bode well.) For four days, fourteen-hours a day, my husband and I sorted, donated, pitched and packed her belongings until everything was ready. Then on the fifth morning, he drove off with a truck full of Mom's possessions and her car in tow - for the thousand mile road trip to Ohio. That same afternoon, Mom walked out of the condo, locked the door behind her, and she and I got into a taxi and rode to the airport. As we drove away, I noticed that she didn't look back.

I guess Mom really did like to travel though, because our flight to Ohio was a delightful adventure. She had often said how much she enjoyed flying and this time was no exception. We weren't able to get seats on the plane together, so she sat in the row right in front of me. And as usual, there was candy in her purse, and today it was Hersey's Chocolate Kisses. So during the entire two hour plane ride, Mom kept passing the kisses back to me, one at a time. Then she'd turn to me and smile and start to laugh. I think the people sitting next to us thought we were crazy. But I loved that time with her. It was our private little joke somehow.

Once we disembarked the airplane, however, Mom's mood immediately changed. She started walking up the exit ramp and then suddenly stopped, as if she didn't know what to do. I took her by the hand and guided her, with a dazed look on her face, through the airport and eventually, to my car. Then we drove to her new home.

It was a cold November day but miraculously, the trees still held their fall colors. I knew the view from Mom's apartment balcony would be stunning and I couldn't wait to show it to show her. When we arrived, we took the elevator up to the twelfth floor and I ushered her into her new apartment. Surprisingly, she didn't say anything. So I slid open the glass doors that led to the balcony and we stepped out into the crisp fall air. Below us, a forest of red, gold and yellow stretched in every direction. It was breathtaking. I waited while she took in the view.

Finally, she said, "It's really beautiful." Then she added, "I want to go home now."

I stood there in shock, trying to comprehend what I had just heard. Suddenly, a wave of exhaustion swept over me as if I hadn't slept in days. We went back inside and I reluctantly telephoned my husband. He had made his way into Georgia after driving non-stop with the van and trailer hitch for twelve hours. He pulled into a rest stop to talk with me and listened to my tale of woe. Then he said, "Ok, tell me what to do."

"Keep going," I said. Then I hung up and told Mom, "We can't go back today. I'm too tired. Let's talk about it in the morning."

Rather than leave her alone in the apartment, I decided to spend the night. I curled up on the floor of her empty guest bedroom and fell sleep. The next morning, my husband arrived with Mom's belongings - and for some reason this cheered her up immensely. To my surprise, she announced that she would stay at the apartment after all and I could go home now...

Thus began two wonderful (if at times trying) years of settling Mom in Ohio, decorating the apartment to her liking and including her in our extended family celebrations. She immediately became a delightful fixture in the lives of our two sons, my husband, his mother and his siblings - and of course, me.

However, I also began to notice more signs of Mom's dementia. At first, I thought it was due to the trauma of relocating and I imagined it would clear up with time. But it didn't. She would seem ok, and then out of the blue, she wasn't. Time and time again there was a decline in some functionality or life skill. But rather than a fast, downhill slide, it was more like a slip and then a plateau, where everything seemed to stabilize. Then another slip and another plateau, a slip and a plateau, almost as if life was fortifying itself for the next plummet. Looking back, I believe there was mercy in all of this, although I didn't recognize it at the time.

As Mom's memory problems increased, I did my best to work around them, not mentioning what I saw and just allowing her to live "independently" in her new home - discreetly transferring one daily task after another from hers to my responsibility. I'm sure at times she knew what was happening. Yet, like myself, she preferred to live in denial. When my husband tried to point out to me where this was headed, I wouldn't hear of it. This was partly because, despite the inevitable changes, one thing didn't change. Mom's desire and ability to appreciate didn't diminish. I witnessed her enjoying little moments like spending time with family, being surprised by a beautiful sunset or devouring a bowl of ice cream. And as her caregiver, I wanted to maintain my optimism that she could continue to enjoy life. Of course, it was up to her to take advantage of those opportunities. And she often did.

Nevertheless, it wasn't long before the admonition that she didn't want "to be a burden" crept into our conversations, always followed by my irritated insistence that she wasn't. I didn't realize at the time that perhaps she had a vague sense of what lay ahead which was compelling her to say those things.

Regrettably, I never asked her exactly what she meant.

Chapter Four: Hospital

(If they act irrationally, there's probably a rational reason.)

The two years after we moved Mom from Florida to Ohio were a whirlwind. I spent much of that time sorting out her financial affairs; purchasing and decorating her apartment (she picked out every item, including the furniture, the kitchen cabinets and window treatments); enlisting her new doctors (who changed and strengthened all her medications…grrr); and integrating her into our extended family.

Unfortunately, Mom was forced to tolerate snowy winters which she hated, and to figure out how to walk to the condominium's mail room to get her mail and then find her way back to her apartment, which for her was no small feat. And although she was cordial and friendly toward her neighbors, she couldn't remember any of their names (or their faces either probably.) So in a lot of ways, taking on such a new situation at that time in her life was much more challenging than I realized.

Another challenge was Mom's noted fear of doctors. Whenever she had a doctor's appointment (which happened more frequently now), I would typically wait until the morning of the appointment to let her know about it so that she wouldn't worry. However, one of those mornings turned out to be one that I will never forget...

It was a snowy morning in mid-December. I called Mom to tell her about her doctor's appointment and immediately, I knew something was terribly wrong. She was trying to talk to me but it sounded like gibberish.

"I'll be right over," I said, and hung up the phone in a panic. Was she having a stroke?

When I got to Mom's apartment, she was in her bathrobe, and still sitting by the phone. She said she felt weak and was having trouble breathing. I looked in her pill box and saw that she hadn't taken her medications in three days, and the recent meals we had delivered to her sat untouched in the frig. So I gave her a set of her medications and a few crackers to eat. Then I phoned the doctor.

"Mom can't come for her appointment today," I told the office nurse. "Something's wrong. What should I do?"

"Take her to the hospital emergency room," came the perfunctory reply. What else could she say? After all, doctors no longer make house calls. My heart sank.

I managed to move Mom to the living room couch and we sat together and stared through the glass balcony doors to the wintry scene outside. I told her the doctor wanted her to go to the hospital. She didn't say a word. Nor did I. I had made up my mind that this was her decision.

After about twenty minutes, she said, "We should go. I'm having trouble breathing."

I said ok.

"You knew I should go, didn't you?" she asked. I told her yes, but that I was waiting for her to say so. She thanked me! Regrettably, this was the last time she would decide her fate until her final day.

I got Mom dressed as best I could. Her feet were so swollen that her shoes wouldn't fit, so I wrangled on two pairs of socks instead. Knowing that she would be mortified if I called an ambulance, I decided to take her to the hospital in our car. My husband arrived with a wheelchair from the condominium lobby and we gingerly got her into it. Then we wheeled her out into the hallway and I reluctantly closed the apartment door behind us, not knowing if she would ever see it again.

When we got to the hospital, the doctor determined that Mom had had a mild heart attack. (However, he never mentioned that she also had congestive heart failure that was causing her body to swell and making it hard for her to breathe. I searched on the internet later to figure that out, but didn't realize at the time that it's also an incurable and ultimately terminal condition.) After a couple of hours of intravenous treatments for her breathing and a hot meal which she devoured, Mom sat up on the edge of the bed and announced that she was ready to go home. We told the doctor.

"She's not going anywhere tonight," the doctor said. "We need to keep her for observation." Mom insisted that she wasn't staying. She said she felt fine and wanted to go home. I listened to this exchange, completely unaware that I had any part to play. Finally, the doctor turned to me and said, "While you decide, I'll get her a room in the cardiac unit." Then he walked out.

Mom and I looked at each other. I told her, like I had in Florida, that maybe we should trust the doctor. In reality, I'd had so little experience with hospitals, I really didn't know if we could simply leave. When Mom had arrived at the hospital, she had signed something called a "Consent to Treatment" or "Patient Consent Form" that all patients must sign. It says in effect, "I voluntarily consent to and authorize the administration and performance of all medical treatment and procedures that may be prescribed and deemed appropriate and necessary." Further down in the document, there's another statement that says, "I understand that I may revoke my consent at any time and that this decision is mine alone."

However, I didn't read that far, or ask for a copy to read later. And no one at the hospital pointed out to me that refusal of treatment was a patient's right.

It was nearly midnight before Mom finally got settled into her hospital room. The IV was dripping in more medicine to keep fluid out of her one lung; and she was hooked up to a heart monitor whose irritating alarm sounded every time she moved in a certain way. They also had a catheter in place so she couldn't get up to go to the bathroom, which, due to the catheterization, she felt like she needed to do every five minutes. And with all of these tubes from the various machines attached to her, the nurse told me it was VERY IMPORTANT that Mom not get out of bed. So I decided to stay in her room overnight and keep vigil. My husband went home, and I curled up on the couch to get some sleep.

As I mentioned before, Mom's mental status, especially her short-term memory, had been declining for some time. At home, occasionally she would call me, upset that she had hidden her purse to "test herself" and couldn't find it. Or we'd go grocery shopping and she'd buy the exact same groceries that were already well-stocked in her kitchen. She no longer wrote her own checks or balanced her checkbook. And her wall calendar was filled with Xs where she kept track of what day it was (thanks to the daily newspaper she had delivered.)

So that first night in the hospital, it's quite possible Mom forgot why she was there. This seemed evident by the fact that she tried to get out of bed twenty-four times (I counted) and each time, I coaxed her to lie back down and told her that everything was going to be ok - but she didn't believe me. At one point, she even accused me of bringing her there to die and that this was all part of a "plan". By morning, we were both exhausted. Such a night should have convinced me that staying in the hospital was a bad idea. Yet, the doctors weren't listening to her and wouldn't discharge her. Why didn't I heed her pleading and just insist? I really don't know. Perhaps I was, once again, scared of not doing the right thing, being accused of elder abuse or being frowned upon by the doctor. The appropriate decision seems obvious now, but it was a real quandary at the time.

In reality, I was trying to do the best I could without anyone to guide me. Although Mom and I had reconnected and become closer in recent years, there continued to be things we never talked about. Looking back, having a mother in her 80's and not knowing her preferences regarding end-of-life care seems crazy, but that was our situation. And Mom may have had earlier heart episodes similar to this one, but if she did, I never knew it. Except for her frequent and sometimes baffling last minute cancellation of our plans for the day, I thought everything was fine. So seeing her suddenly in this medical crisis, compounded by the revelation of her fragile mental state which she had artfully concealed (with my willing denial), put me in a state of shock - and I didn't have my bearings to clearly navigate the situation.

For the next four days, Mom never left her bed (although she tried countless times) and I never left the hospital and rarely left her side. I did my best to comfort her, but it didn't help. The longer she stayed, the worse things got. She forgot how to walk, she became withdrawn and weak, she stopped eating and hardly spoke. Having never heard of or seen a person with hospital delirium, I mistakenly blamed Mom's worsening state on her medical condition rather than on the hospital stay itself. And her doctors did the same. Tragically, she was stuck on a three-foot by seven-foot island with no sign of rescue in sight.

Slowly, the fluid in Mom's body started to build up again and the doctors increased her IV treatments. One night, during another dangerous episode of shortness of breath, I asked the attending doctor about hospice, hoping to ease some of her pain and suffering. He thought it was appropriate to consider, and said that he would schedule a consultation. I didn't know what a consultation would involve, who would be there or when it would happen. My main concern was why the decision couldn't be made right then, while she was in this state. But I didn't ask any of this.

The next day, my husband and my younger son were visiting with Mom. As I tried to feed her some lunch, she suddenly started shouting that she wanted all this to end and she wanted someone to do something about it. It seemed like she was trying to get them to listen to her. Because Mom was declining so fast, I thought maybe she meant she wanted to dispense with all her medical treatments so she could die in peace. I ran and got the doctor on call and brought her back to Mom's room. I asked Mom to repeat to the doctor what she had told me and she started shouting at the doctor, "I want to live! I want to live!"

Looking back, it's obvious now that Mom was saying, "Get me out of here! Get me out of here!" However, at that moment, I was totally confused. Was she still capable of making her own decisions? Or as her health care proxy, was I now the decision maker? I had brought along the Durable Power of Attorney for Health Care document and it was on record at the hospital if I needed it. However, if this was the time, what decisions was I supposed to be making? Medical decisions for Mom as I saw them or upholding her decisions about herself? If you had asked me then, I would have given a different answer than I would give now.

The doctor pulled me aside and said, "It's all about her now. No issues between you and her - and no guilt." I had no idea what she meant but somehow I felt I was being blamed for something. Then the doctor said that it was premature to talk about hospice and she wouldn't recommend it, and she walked out. (I now know that it is not uncommon for physicians to postpone approving hospice until the patient has three months or less to live. . .Mom died exactly three months after my conversation with this doctor.)

Shortly after all this, Mom's mental fog lifted a bit. She started eating and talking again, and after seven days in the hospital the doctors decided to discharge her - to rehabilitation therapy. This new development totally surprised me, since Mom had been fairly functional before she arrived at the E.R. and she didn't have any surgeries or falls in the hospital that would have warranted physical therapy. So why did she need to go to rehab? Evidently, those seven days in the hospital were so traumatic for her that she was now rendered an invalid who needed professional help to regain some of her functionality. (Sadly, despite going through therapy, Mom would never regain her ability to walk unassisted.)

A hospital social worker came to Mom's room to advise us. Unfortunately, she didn't mention home therapy as an option, so I chose to send Mom to the rehabilitation wing of an assisted living facility that was near her apartment, although I had never seen its rehab area. In fact, I had no clue what a rehab facility was or that it meant Mom was just moving from one type of hospital setting (acute care) to another (sub-acute care).

On her last night in the hospital, the nurses tried to change Mom's IV needle to avoid switching her to oral medication. The nurse stuck Mom's arm twelve times and then gave up because her veins were so brittle. Had the nurse documented this in Mom's medical record, it could have potentially prevented her from being stuck unnecessarily in the future. Instead, I was told simply that the doctor determined Mom could take her meds by mouth after all. Oh.

But we weren't out of the woods yet. The next day, the rehab facility called and said they wanted Mom's catheter changed before she could be transferred. Sometimes catheters are needed, but often they are implemented for staff convenience so the patient doesn't need to use the bathroom. Three nurses came into Mom's room to do the deed and hold her down during the procedure - and I was told to leave the room. However, I could hear Mom screaming from the other side of the door so I went back in and refused the procedure.

To my surprise, they stopped.

Chapter Five: Rehab

(Assisted Living doesn't necessarily assist.)

Three days before Christmas, Mom was finally leaving the hospital cardiac unit where she had been sequestered for eight straight days. Although it was nearly nine o'clock at night, an ambulance transported her to the skilled nursing unit of an assisted living facility that I had picked out for her to do her rehab.

Thankfully, the ambulance ride turned out to be a somewhat cheery occasion for Mom because the emergency medical technicians were in a holiday mood and had hung Christmas lights and a miniature Christmas tree inside the back of the ambulance - which she enjoyed immensely. When we arrived at the facility, I walked behind her as she was wheeled by gurney to the back of the assisted living building and then up the elevator to the rehabilitation wing. After we entered the unit, the door automatically slammed shut and locked behind us, and I was told that this was a combination Alzheimer/Rehab floor and was always in lock-down. (In other words, it was the closest thing to being in prison without really being in one.)

Evidently, the residents were already asleep in their rooms, except for a few poor souls who sat slumped over tables in the common area, their heads buried in their arms. We were led past them to the private room that I had reserved for Mom and when I saw it, I was shocked. It had bare, dingy-white walls and a single lightbulb in the ceiling. What happened to the nice decor I once saw in the assisted living area??

The nurse on duty seemed perturbed about getting an admission so late at night, and that Mom didn't have a catheter, so I volunteered to spend the night (thinking I'd look for another rehab facility in the morning). I draped a blanket over the well-worn La-Z-Boy chair next to Mom's bed and tried to get some sleep...Admittedly, this place gave me the creeps.

It was another restless night. Mom got up a few times and I took her to the bathroom. Now that the catheter was out, she did ok. However, she needed a wheelchair to navigate because she had forgotten how to walk. At least, she wasn't tethered to all those cords and tubes like in the hospital! The next morning, I decided Mom would stay here after all (and so would I). I hoped that her mental issues would subside now that she was in a slightly less hectic medical environment. I was also concerned that moving her again might make things worse.

Unfortunately, I didn't realize the importance of the social and environmental cues that Mom had established at her apartment so she could function. As I've mentioned, her daily newspaper told her what day it was. She wrote herself notes like "Don't wear the purple pants again" so she wouldn't repeat certain things. And then there was her external identity - her wig, her wedding rings, her purse - that I took from her for safekeeping when she entered the hospital. She didn't even have a mirror to look at herself! Unbeknownst to me, it was the absence of these things in the sterile environment of the hospital and now the rehab facility that laid bare how poor her short-term memory actually was.

Another issue was that the rehab staff had labeled Mom a "high fall risk" because she couldn't walk and yet she had a propensity to try to get out of bed. The ways to address this were either to tether her to the bed with arm restraints or to place a mat under her mattress that sounded an alarm when she got up. The first option wasn't an option of course, and the second option didn't work. The alarm would sound for a good fifteen minutes before anyone came to check on her. So for two weeks, I camped out in Mom's room twenty-four hours a day and basically became the safety net to keep her from falling. (One night, I tried sleeping at home and the next day a nurse told me that Mom had fallen during the night but she assured me that Mom hadn't hurt herself.)

Mom's therapy sessions started the morning after she arrived and I went along. Her first task was to start using a walker. Mom had always been thin, but today she looked extremely frail, and I noticed how much effort it took for her just to follow the therapist's instructions. Besides being in a weakened state, she obviously had no idea of where she was or why she was doing all this.

Two days into the therapy sessions, the staff wouldn't let me go with her anymore, so Mom refused to go at all. And when Mom decided not to do something, there was no point in trying to talk her into it. The therapist gave me a strong warning that if Mom continued to refuse therapy, Medicare might not pay for her stay. I had no idea what she was talking about because I didn't know anything about Medicare and I hadn't even thought about the cost of all this or who was paying for it. But I did know that Mom's health was not improving, and as the days went by she seemed to be getting worse.

I tried to persuade her to go to the common area for activities but she wasn't interested. I begged her to let me take her for a stroll in the wheelchair, but she refused. She wouldn't leave her room and only got out of bed when they made her do so for meals (which she hardly ate) or to use the bathroom. She was quiet and she seemed depressed or preoccupied, and I was worried about her.

Late one night, as I sat in the common area watching tv, a nurse came up to me and asked how I thought Mom was doing. I told her I didn't know, but it didn't seem good. "I think she belongs in hospice," she whispered to me. "Don't tell anyone I said so. I'm not supposed to bring this up. I'd give her three months," she added. As I watched her go off to her patient rounds, I considered what she had said. It confirmed to me that what I was observing about Mom was truly serious. And I now knew for certain that the medical staff was not going to bring up hospice unless I did.

The next day, I asked the physician's assistant about hospice. She said I would need a second doctor's opinion to approve it. For some reason, it didn't occur to me to ask for the resident doctor (whom I hadn't met yet) and it wasn't suggested. So I scheduled an appointment for Mom to be transported back to the hospital in a few days to see a local authority on congestive heart failure. It seemed that a terminal diagnosis of congestive heart failure was our only chance to get her out of this medical experiment that her life had become. Unfortunately, I didn't realize that I could take her home at anytime. I still wasn't sure of my rights as her health care proxy or hers as the patient.

However, we never made it to that appointment. The day after my conversation with the physician's assistant, it was Mom's birthday. Mom asked me how old she was. "Eighty-seven," I told her proudly. She stared at her birthday cards and said nothing. I could tell that at this juncture in her illness, she was slipping away. I knew she didn't want to be in an institution. And she hated and feared procedures and doctors. It clearly wasn't her intention to live as an invalid - and as she constantly reminded me, she didn't want to be a burden.

So, two days later, when the unexpected happened, I felt ok about it.

Chapter Six: Time to Go

(Not all medical advice is good advice.)

Two days after Mom's eighty-seventh birthday was a frigid winter's day. Her room at the rehab facility was growing dark in the early dusk and the solitary light bulb in the ceiling waited expectantly but no one thought to turn it on - because something extremely important was happening in the bed before us. Mom lay on her back, eyes closed, breathing softly and rapidly and sleeping. She looked relaxed and peaceful, as if all the anxiety and fear of recent weeks had drained from her face. It was a relief to see her like that. This was the mom I remembered. Even at her advanced age, she looked beautiful.

My older son sat at one side of her bed, his youthful frame silhouetted by the wintry scene outside the window. On a whim, he had brought his guitar and was playing it softly in the shadows. It was the perfect accompaniment to what was happening, giving Mom something sweet and gentle to focus on and conveying our unspoken permission if she wanted to go.

I sat at Mom's other side, in the same La-Z-Boy chair that had been my makeshift bed for the past two weeks. I held her hand and alternated between gazing at her face and staring out the window. I didn't say anything. There was nothing to say. She had been through so much and it had been so hard to watch. We had been on this journey together and now all was well. She might be leaving us. Yet, it seemed so sweet somehow. She was comfortable - and so was I. It was a pivotal moment.

My main concern was not to disturb her. As if by some miracle, the nursing staff had failed to check on us for hours, so we had had this precious time to spend with Mom - time to reflect, time to love, time to appreciate.

Then, I made a huge mistake.

A nurse aide came in and I casually mentioned to her what was happening. She immediately ran out and got the physician's assistant. The physician's assistant rushed in, took one look at Mom and with great concern declared that she wanted to do a chest x- ray and a urine sample. This was so surprising and out of sync with what we were witnessing that I felt a shock wave run through me. Why the sudden intrusion? Somehow, it didn't seem right. This was lovely and peaceful. Mom did not appear to be in any pain. We were content to let her pass in peace. Why did we have to do all this? But the physician's assistant convinced me that the tests were just routine and that they wouldn't disturb her. So I said ok, not knowing where this was headed.

The tests determined that Mom had pneumonia and a serious urinary tract infection. Evidently, these two maladies are quite common among elderly patients in skilled nursing facilities and often account for their short lifespan once they are admitted. The physician's assistant recommended sending her to the hospital. It was eight o'clock at night and I knew Mom didn't want the whole hospital thing again, but I wasn't thinking clearly. I was physically and emotionally exhausted from our rollercoaster ride of the last three weeks. So I said that I didn't want any invasive procedures done (although I really had no idea what that meant at the time.) She assured me that they would just give Mom antibiotics at the hospital and it wouldn't cause her any pain. I felt pressured to make a decision, so I said, "If she was your mother, what would you do?"

"I would go to the hospital," the physician's assistant replied, "So that when she does die it will not be due to infection and she will be more comfortable."

Looking back, I know now that that answer didn't make any sense. Mom wasn't in any pain and she seemed completely comfortable. It seemed like they wanted Mom out of the facility to prevent her from dying under their watch - but I didn't know why. Unfortunately, I did not have the confidence I needed as her health care proxy to refuse any further intervention. If I'd had my wits about me, I would have demanded to talk with the attending physician, whom I had not met in the two weeks that we'd been in rehab. Supposedly, he had been sick with the flu the whole time, although it was during the Christmas holidays, so who knows? Anyway, there was no way he was coming in tonight, they said. So I didn't insist. I gave in and said ok. The physician's assistant immediately gave Mom a shot in her buttocks and called for an ambulance.

Emergency medical technicians arrived and wheeled Mom outside into the single-digit weather. I jumped into the front seat of the ambulance and thought we would be going right away, but one of the technicians told me that before we left she wanted to start an IV.

I told her, "Her veins have been collapsing, she's been stuck so much. I'd like you to wait."

No reply.

So I sat for ten minutes while the back of the ambulance stood wide open (and Mom lay there with pneumonia) until the attendant finally slammed the door shut in frustration.

"Did you do it?" I asked.

"No. They collapsed."

STUPID.

As we rode in the ambulance to a different hospital this time, I thought about what had happened during Mom's first hospital stay two weeks earlier. I could only hope that this experience would be better.

Could it be any worse???

Chapter Seven: Moving, Again

(Necessity is the mother of invention.)

After just twelve days in rehab, and a sweet near-departing, Mom was in a hospital for the second time in a month. I was kicking myself for agreeing to this. Why were we here? Somehow it felt wrong. Immediately, another IV was inserted into her arm, and the heavy-duty antibiotics began to work. Soon she awoke from her deep state of leaving us as if she had been in a dream - and she looked at me and smiled. I had never seen her look so peaceful.

"My little Lindy," she said, and she squeezed my hand.

Twenty-four hours later, her appetite was good and she seemed to be bouncing back a bit from the pneumonia. However, in addition to the antibiotics, she was once again receiving diuretic drugs because she still had congestive heart failure and fluid was building up in her lung. Added to this, she now was receiving oxygen 24-hours a day, with a tube running from her nose to a compressor machine nearby. Despite my pleadings, the Med/Surg doctor and the cardiologist refused to approve her for hospice. Instead, they agreed to order palliative care. I had no idea what palliative care was, but it didn't seem to change the situation at all except for discontinuing a few of her routine meds.

One thing that did become obvious though was how much the nurses in the hospital relied on me to take care of Mom. I was there day and night, and at one point when I left her for a few minutes to track down a vending machine and scrounge something to eat, a nurse met me when I got back and proceeded to chastise me for leaving Mom alone. She caught her trying to get out of bed, she said. What is their job anyway, I wondered?

After another three-day stint of confining Mom to her bed, the hospital finally decided to discharge her back to the rehab facility. Before we left, the nurse came in and disconnected her IV, but said she wanted to insert a more permanent (PICC) line to deliver Mom's antibiotics. I didn't know what a PICC line was, but it sounded invasive. Against my better judgment and with the nurse's insistence, I said ok without asking what the procedure entailed. I was told to stay out of Mom's room while they did it, and three nurses worked on Mom for over twenty minutes. When they finally came out, one of the nurses said they weren't successful and wanted to try again. I told them absolutely not - and they left.

At the last minute, before Mom could leave the hospital, the doctor ordered an echocardiogram. Again, I said no to this, but the nurses convinced me that it was just to get a picture and it wouldn't be invasive. Mom was brought down into the basement of the hospital and we waited in a hallway for half an hour before we were finally brought in for the scan. Then the tech spent nearly an hour searching for Mom's heart (which he couldn't find and didn't get the pictures he wanted anyway.) The worst part was Mom had to pee and was forced to use a bed pan during the procedure, which thoroughly embarrassed her. I felt so bad about it.

It was evening before Mom was finally transported back to her old room at the rehab facility. My husband agreed to start spending the night in the LazyBoy chair next to her bed because I was so sleep deprived I just couldn't do it any more. From then on, he stayed with her each night and I stayed with her during the day. Once again, she refused to go to her therapy sessions, and she still frequently got up from bed (or tried to). The one new addition to her situation was that now she had a tube under her nose for oxygen and since the oxygen tubing followed her everywhere, it was an additional fall risk factor.

Three more days passed, and now Mom seemed more alert. One afternoon, I took her for a long stroll in her wheelchair and she seemed to really enjoy it. At one point, she said, "Don't give up on me." I said I wouldn't. But I knew I could never do the hospital thing again. Not with her dementia. It would be too much for both of us.

A day later, after living in Mom's room for almost a month, we finally met the rehab facility doctor for the first time. We watched him sign Mom's "Do Not Resuscitate" order and it dawned on us that this was why the physician's assistant had frantically wanted Mom to go to the hospital when she contracted pneumonia. The doctor also told us that pneumonia used to be called the "old people's best friend" because it was such a peaceful way to die. I won't write here what I was thinking when he told me that. But it just confirmed to my husband and I that after a month of being in rehab facilities and hospitals, it was time to get Mom out of there. Besides the risk of infection, it just seemed better and easier to care for her at home. And lo and behold, when we told the nurse of our plans, the rehab social worker suddenly appeared with information about home rehabilitation.

So we enlisted a home health care service and rented a hospital bed, a portable commode, an oxygen compressor, a wheelchair, and a walker. I selected a home health care doctor who I thought we could work with and he agreed to keep Mom on palliative care. I set up Mom's physical and occupational therapy home visits and bought her a wardrobe of stretchy pajama pants because her clothes no longer fit due to her increasing congestive heart failure water weight. And we got the largest slippers we could find to cover her swollen feet.

Our spare room became Mom's bedroom and we added a recliner for my husband to sleep on. He had agreed to continue keeping vigil by Mom's bed at night so she wouldn't fall if she tried to get up. I was beyond appreciative. I knew Mom's health was extremely fragile and it seemed impossible that she could ever live independently again. Therefore, we had no idea what the future held.

All I knew was that for now, Mom was coming home with us.

Chapter Eight: Home Caring

(Who they are at the end is not necessarily who they are.)

After her second hospital stay and seven more days in rehab (they didn't even try to make her do therapy this time), we were finally taking Mom home. The temperature outside had been in single digits for weeks, so we waited for the first sunny day where the mercury rose above freezing to transport her to our house. When I told Mom about the move, she put up a fuss. She said she liked where she was and she wasn't going anywhere. This was sadly amusing because if someone had asked her where she was or why she was there, she couldn't have told them.

I explained to her that she couldn't stay at the rehab facility because she refused to do her physical therapy and besides, we could take better care of her at home. I now know that my response probably sounded like a rebuke, as the strain of caregiving was once again creeping into our conversations. (Unfortunately, I didn't realize it at the time.) Despite her resistance, we put Mom in a wheelchair, steered her out to my car and drove to our house. When we got there she couldn't walk, of course, so my husband picked her up, wheelchair and all, and carried her up our front steps - and there she was.

Almost immediately, we settled into a routine of doling out her daily meds and keeping track of her oxygen. My husband (who's a great cook) cooked all her meals and everything appeared to be ok. However, Mom was very sick, and it didn't seem likely that she would ever get better. Her body was quite swollen from the congestive heart failure, and she was extremely weak. When the physician's assistant came for his first home visit (why did we so rarely see a doctor?), I again brought up the subject of hospice. He said he thought Mom would probably qualify and he'd be back in two weeks to check on her.

However, something else was going on with Mom. Since her near death experience with pneumonia, she had begun acting delusional again, much like she had during her first time in the hospital - but this was much worse. After we moved her into our house, she started lashing out at me at night and she seemed almost gripped by fear. We still needed someone to be with her at all times, so I did my best to keep her calm when I was with her. Pretty soon, though, my husband took over most of her care because I worried that I might be making things worse. I don't know how he was able to do it. Her ups and downs were hard to watch, much less manage. Mom would gain water weight, which would cause her to struggle to breathe and she'd appear to be failing; then she'd get better; then she'd get worse. I finally called the physician's assistant and told him what was happening. He said he would order a hospice evaluation.

Miraculously, ten days later, Mom's health had slowly improved - sort of. Her water weight was down, she was making effort with her in-home physical therapy sessions and she seemed steadier on her feet. It even looked like she might soon be able to walk a bit without her walker. Perhaps she will live for a long time, I thought, or possibly move back to her own apartment. Yet at night, she continued to have nightmares and the focus of her suspicions was on me. When I came downstairs each morning, she would be sitting at the breakfast table, whispering to my husband that I had come into her room the previous night and threatened her. Or if we were sitting alone together, she would glare at me and say repeatedly, "Why do you hate me?" I would try to tell her I didn't hate her, I loved her, but my insistence was futile.

Like a perfect storm, the weather wasn't helping either. We were having a record cold and snowy winter, so Mom was cooped up in the house day and night. I yearned to take her for a walk. One day, out of desperation, I opened the front door and let her sit in the doorway for a while. It seemed to help clear her mind. At one point, she turned to me and said, "You've had a hard time, haven't you? I'm sorry for all this." Words can't describe how much it meant to hear her say that.

When the physician's assistant came for his second visit, he examined Mom and decided she was doing too well to qualify for hospice. I had to admit that physically she seemed to be better. But otherwise things kept getting crazier. She wanted to sleep by the front door at night because she thought someone was trying to get in. And she was totally paranoid about me. On the one hand I knew it was just her disease, but soon my health was being affected. I started getting headaches and toothaches, and I began to feel like an unwelcome guest in my own home. This left me sad and heartbroken. I had given my all to help her and now I had become her mortal enemy!

I realized, of course, that part of my reaction to the situation was due to my home life when I was growing up. Dad never hit Mom or me, but shouting matches and tirades were a matter of course. So now Mom's delirious attacks, regardless of its cause, brought back my childhood feelings of wanting to flee or escape. And it was something I just couldn't shake. I finally told my husband that if Mom's condition stabilized and she began to walk without her walker, then we needed to move her back to her apartment.

One night, in an attempt to speed up the process and relieve me of my mental anguish, my husband decided to see if Mom could walk on her own. He asked her to take a few steps without her walker and she did - and then she fell. It was a very scary moment. And a defining one. I tried not to show my disappointment, but I was so miserable, I realized right then that either Mom or I would have to go. What a heart-wrenching realization that I could no longer be with my own mother!

So my husband offered to move Mom back to her apartment and take care of her there. (What husband does this, right?) As much as I didn't want this to happen, I saw no other choice. The next day, I watched as he loaded her into his car and drove away, and I thought about how Mom had been in our home for only fifteen days and already she was being forced to leave.

Had I failed? I don't know. I can only say I felt relief.

Chapter Nine: Back Home Again

(Despite our best efforts, things happen.)

After spending two weeks in our home and failing to "qualify" for hospice, Mom was back at her apartment and my husband was taking care of her there. At night, he slept on the floor outside her bedroom to keep vigil because she was still waking up delirious and afraid. He said that at first she talked about witches, but eventually things got better.

Now that Mom was out of our house, I felt some stress relief and was able to visit with her during the day. On one of my visits, she had difficulty breathing and complained of chest pains. Was this another heart attack? I gave her some heart medicine and that seemed to help. Yet, the episode reminded me of just how fragile she was - indeed, anything could happen at any moment.

Eventually, I had to explain to the physician's assistant why we moved Mom back to her apartment, and he prescribed her an anti-psychotic drug, which seemed like an extreme measure and I hesitated to use it. Then one evening, as I was putting Mom to bed, she had another twilight meltdown and accused me of sneaking into the apartment and harassing her. The venom in her words caught me off guard and totally devastated me, and I vowed right then and there that I couldn't be with her again until her paranoia diminished. That's when my husband tried giving her the anti-psychotic medication - but it didn't help. I finally told him that if she asked, to say that I had gone on a business trip. I hoped that she would just forget I existed.

Still, I was desperate to know why Mom was attacking me, so I arranged for a psychologist to come to the apartment and do an evaluation. My husband said that Mom asked the psychologist, "Did my daughter put you up to this?" and that the examination was extremely distressful for her. Plus, it also proved to be a fairly big waste of time. The one thing I learned was that Mom had very little short term memory. How does a person function without a short-term memory? In this case, I guess it was both a blessing and a curse. It allowed her to forget the pain of her predicament, but she also wasn't able to understand why she was in that predicament in the first place. I was also told that she might have a combination of Alzheimer's and vascular dementia, although there was no explanation of why those chronic diseases worsened so severely during her first hospitalization and again after her second.

Physically though, Mom seemed to be making great progress. My husband reported to me that she was walking further and further with her walker; she didn't need her oxygen for hours at a time; and he was giving her less and less of the diuretic drug because her water weight had begun to stabilize. Eventually, he was able to stop the diuretic altogether and amazingly, Mom stopped hallucinating. (Was this a coincidence or were delusions a possible side effect of the drug, I wondered?) At any rate, after two weeks of not seeing her, I decided it was time to return.

We had imagined that Mom's home therapy might go on for months, but she was doing so well, the occupational and physical therapists soon discharged her and the home care nurse came for a final visit. Unfortunately, the nurse arrived complaining of a nasty stomach flu - and within two days, Mom had it as well. So even though Mom had "graduated" from home therapy, the flu took its toll and soon she wasn't nearly as strong as she had been just a few days earlier. She couldn't walk as far with her walker. She needed her oxygen far more often. And no matter what we tried or the doctor prescribed, she couldn't shake that stubborn stomach flu.

In the midst of all this, we had to put Mom back on the diuretic medication because her water weight began to creep up again. Before long, she was staying up most of night and sleeping most of the day. When I asked her why she didn't sleep at night, she answered, "Because it's more interesting at night." Oh boy, what did that mean? She was probably experiencing hallucinations again, but thankfully, she didn't mention it to me. So I too moved into the apartment to help take care of her.

At that point, either my husband or I had been by Mom's side constantly for about three months. One day, she asked why one of us was always with her. I couldn't bring myself to say, "Because you can't be left alone." It would have broken my heart to say that. So I explained that it was because she took off her oxygen tubing and didn't put it back on, and she needed it, which was true. Mom would often follow the tubing around the apartment or gather it up in her hands and ask, "What is this thing? Why am I wearing this?" And then she would take it off and leave it somewhere.

Nevertheless, our present caregiving arrangement didn't answer two looming questions, "What's going to happen to Mom?" and "What are we going to do?" Something had to be decided because my husband and I were running out of steam, both physically and emotionally. We couldn't continue to live at her apartment and I wasn't mentally ready to move her back to our house. So we started looking for alternatives - and soon, regrettably, we got our answers...

It all began the day I went to tour a new assisted living facility. This one had a nurse's station on every floor and a doctor on call, yet it looked classy and felt more like a normal apartment building than an institution. Looking back, I don't know what I was thinking. From every indication Mom had made in the past, she would never have wanted to live there. However, we were desperate to find a solution and her physician's assistant told us he didn't think she needed to be in a memory care unit (which both surprised and delighted us), so this place seemed ideal. Plus, the cost was less than half of what around-the-clock private duty home care in her apartment would have been, so I signed the contract that very day and put down a deposit.

I knew Mom had been fretting about what was going to happen to her, so when I got back to the apartment, I enthusiastically told her about this new place and showed her pictures. She seemed pleased. That night, as I tucked her into bed, I thought about her question of why we were always with her. I decided that rather than camping out in the living room to keep an eye on her nighttime wanderings, as we usually did, tonight we would sleep in the guest bedroom so she could have some privacy if she wanted to explore her apartment a bit.

My husband was fast asleep when I heard the thump of Mom's walker as she went past our bedroom door. Keeping to my plan, I decided not to follow her. Besides, I knew if I put her back to bed she would just get up again and this was her only opportunity for a little solitude and freedom. As she passed by, I peeked in the hallway and saw that the oxygen tubing had followed her into the kitchen. Good. I could hear her rummaging through drawers and opening cabinets and then checking the front door lock. After about fifteen minutes, I heard the thump of the walker again as she headed back to her room.

A few moments later there was a loud thud. My husband and I both leapt out of bed at the same time and we found Mom sprawled out on the floor of her bedroom, the walker standing a few steps away. Evidently, she had reached her bedroom closet without using it and had fallen as she tried to get back to bed. Now, her hip was killing her and she couldn't get up.

It was one a.m. and I knew she (and we) were exhausted. So I decided to let her rest where she was. I had no idea what lie ahead, but something told me this was going to be a very, very long day. I covered up Mom with a blanket and laid down on the floor beside her.

Then we both fell asleep.

Chapter Ten: 'Til the Final Day

(The more intense it gets, the more likely the end is near.)

It had been just three weeks since my husband moved Mom back to her apartment. Now she had fallen - and when she and I awoke on the floor of her bedroom, it was 4 a.m. Even though she was in a lot of pain, we somehow got her into her wheelchair and called 911. Then the emergency medical technicians arrived and checked her over. At first, they thought she might be ok - but eventually they decided to take her to a hospital in their ambulance.

When we arrived at the hospital, the orthopedic surgeon confirmed that Mom had broken her hip and he recommended surgery right away. My first response was "No." I had told myself many times that I would not put her through the hospital experience again. I had to stand my ground.

However, the surgeon's justifications sounded compelling. He explained that without the surgery she would never walk again, she might be in a lot of pain for the rest of her life, and she couldn't live as long with a broken hip. I called Mom's home care physician's assistant and told him I didn't want to put Mom through the surgery. He concurred with the hospital that she should have the operation. I hung up the phone, knowing the surgeon was waiting for my decision. It felt like I didn't have much time to think.

In retrospect, I should have demanded a hospice consultation right then and there. Here was an eighty-seven year old woman with one lung, on continuous oxygen, suffering from a worsening chronic and terminal illness (congestive heart failure), prone to infections, and living with debilitating dementia and delirium. She had had four hospital and/or rehab stays in the last twelve weeks. She had no short-term memory and, at best, was bound to a walker before she fell, plus she required constant supervision because she remained a serious fall risk. And with this proposed surgery, she was facing a protracted stint in a rehabilitation facility which she had already demonstrated she was incapable of completing successfully.

I don't know what the outcome of the hospice consultation would have been, but perhaps there was a chance that a voice of sanity from the medical community would have backed me up and said, "Let her live out her days in peace." As it was, there was no such voice. Even Mom's primary care physician, who had been our family doctor for over twenty-five years, never once called me to follow up on her situation after my frantic phone call to his office three months earlier. I had traveled this medical nightmare without a doctor's support, and now the hospitalist was pushing for a decision. Unfortunately, trusting the hospitalist's advice rather than my gut instinct had become my default in Mom's journey. So I said to go ahead.

I held Mom's hand as they took her into the surgery prep area, then I was told to leave. As I left her side, she started yelling for me. She was so scared. I saw them put an oxygen mask over her face as she struggled to talk. She had no idea what was going on. It was awful. When I finally got to see her in the Recovery Room, she was lying there unconscious, with an intubation tube stuck down her throat and a ventilator machine making her breathe - all routine procedures, I was told, when someone requires general anesthesia during surgery. I must admit that the nurse who told me this didn't sound very convincing.

After her operation, Mom was kept in the Intensive Care Unit for two days. We didn't stay with her because she was supposedly being watched constantly by the nursing staff. However, I discovered that the nurses were giving her sleeping pills because they claimed that she was "restless." Basically, they were drugging her. And if Mom took one of those pills, she was knocked out and groggy for most of the following day. It was really weird to see her like that.

When she was finally moved to the Orthopedic Surgery ward, my husband began staying with her at night again and I stayed with her during the day, because I just couldn't do the night shift anymore. Like the previous times, Mom was catheterized (hooked up to a urine bag so she couldn't go pee or feel when she needed to) and she continued to get intravenous medications. And of course, there was an air compressor cycling on and off constantly to supply her with twenty-four hour oxygen. She also had inflatable cuffs on her legs to keep her blood from clotting and she was told not to put any weight on her left hip.

Of course, there was also the one thing that Mom hated the most. She wasn't allowed to get out of bed and she kept trying to do so. To address this situation at night, the nurse wanted to give her another sleeping pill. We explained how groggy Mom acted the next day after taking those. So the nurse gave her half of a pill instead. That was almost as bad. My husband said Mom woke up in the middle of the night, totally disoriented and terrified.

It was during her second evening in the Orthopedic Surgery ward that Mom confided in my husband that she felt really blue, and she began to cry. My husband called me and begged me to come to the hospital. I was so burnt out, I told him I couldn't - but he sounded desperate, so I went anyway. When I got to the hospital, Mom was sitting on the edge of her bed, looking very distraught. She said she felt like something really bad was going to happen to her and she couldn't shake it. Did I know what it was? I said no, I didn't. She said my eyes looked sad.

And then she said:

"If you speak up, they think you're a problem.
If you laugh, they think you're silly.
If you keep quiet, they think you're an imbecile."

This was such a profound observation, it almost startled me. I finally saw what little quality of life Mom now had. She kept saying over and over, "What are we doing here? Why are we here? (And five minutes later) What are we waiting for?" She had no recollection of her hip surgery. She didn't know why she was commanded to stay in bed. She not only didn't know where she was, she didn't know *who* she was, and she kept checking the hospital ID band on her wrist as if it was the only reference to her identity.

As I looked at Mom, I thought of that fateful night at the rehab facility only three months earlier, when she almost passed away from pneumonia. I recalled my conversation with the physician's assistant, declaring to her that I didn't want any further invasive treatments and asking what she would do if this were her mother. And I remembered her response, "If she were my mother, I would send her to the hospital so that when she does die, it will not be due to infection and she will be more comfortable." Was this her idea of "more comfortable"?

The next day, Mom said something with such finality that it almost took my breath away. Looking back, I realized there were many times during her two years in Ohio when she and I would make plans for the day and then, at the last moment, she'd cancel them. At the time, I didn't know why this was happening and I found it a bit irritating. However, now I began to understand that she must have had moments when she didn't feel well or she felt like something bad might happen to her. Yet, she hid her medical symptoms from me because she didn't want to pursue them. So on this day, after all she had been through, she said to me, or actually she didn't really even say it to me - she just said this,

> "I knew this was going to happen."

It was as if all those opportunities for denial that had helped her cope with life's difficulties in the past had finally run out. Here she was, a human being who didn't know what was going on or where she was, with an overwhelming sense of impending doom. She was finally up against a wall that couldn't be ignored or wished away and she knew it. How tragic is that?

Five days after her hip surgery, the surgeon told us that we could once again move Mom to a rehab facility. My husband and I resolved not to go back to the same place as before, so I made an appointment with the hospital's social worker to ask for suggestions. She said she wasn't allowed to make any facility recommendations. And still no one talked to us about hospice.

I knew of another assisted living place that had a rehab unit. I sent my husband to look at it and he said that it looked nice. There was a semi-private room available right across from the nurses' station, which was important so someone could keep an eye on Mom. And there was already a patient in the room, so Mom would have some company. I checked with the social worker and she said the place was new and that there were no complaints thus far. So we decided to move Mom there.

Before the hospital could transport her, however, the rehab facility required that Mom have a bowel movement, so the nurse gave her a stool softener. When it didn't work, she gave her an extra dose. I was completely unfamiliar with stool softeners. All I knew was that the nurse kept us waiting and waiting, and when the medication still didn't work by evening, she sent for the ambulance anyway. For some reason, Mom was always being transported when her paranoia was at its worst. And tonight, she was more fearful than I had ever seen her. She begged me not to let her leave the hospital. She was really hysterical. I held her hand all the way to the ambulance and while they loaded her into the back of the van. Then I climbed into the front passenger seat.

The cab was separated from the back of the ambulance this time, so I couldn't see Mom and she couldn't see me. And the ambulance ride seemed to take forever. The driver was in a chatty mood and didn't seem to be in any hurry to get to our destination. He took a longer route to the rehab facility and got stuck in rush-hour traffic, so by the time we arrived it was after 6 p.m. Mom was beyond freaked and her blood pressure was 160/110. On top of this, there was no oxygen compressor set up in her room and the ambulance driver took his oxygen tanks with him. So we waited nearly twenty minutes for Mom's oxygen set up to arrive, and while we were waiting, her oxygen saturation dropped to 72 percent, which was dangerously low.

The rehab facility also wouldn't give Mom a bedside commode, although she was fresh from hip surgery, because the physical therapist who needed to evaluate her had already gone for the day. Supposedly, Mom would be evaluated first thing in the morning. In the meantime, she would need to be carried to the bathroom by a male nurse. Why I didn't raise holy hell about this, I'll never know.

As if on cue, the stool softener finally started to work, so the male nurse carried Mom into the bathroom and set her on the commode. I went in with her. It was so embarrassing for her. She had a sort of diarrhea episode and because she had been carried, her hip was now killing her. She told me, "I've never experienced such pain." Then she said, "Llee, I don't think I'm going to make it." What could I say? I told her that we'd have to do the best that we could. She said ok.

The nurse brought in all the legal forms and I signed them, including the "Do Not Resuscitate" order. Learning from my past experience, I asked when that form would be signed by the doctor and he assured me that it would be signed within 24 hours. Mom was put back in bed and they brought her her dinner. She ate a few bites and was pleasant but quiet. I asked if she liked her room. She said yes. I asked if she was in pain. She said no. I noticed "Wheel of Fortune" was on the TV but she wasn't watching it.

Then I did something that I truly regret. I got a phone call from a friend and I took it in Mom's room. The friend asked me how Mom was doing and I said, "We think she is doing OK, but she's just had hip surgery and she's gaining all this water weight again and blowing up like a balloon." Here I was, talking about Mom as if she wasn't there - and I didn't even realize it.

Unfortunately, the patient who was supposed to share Mom's room had been transferred. And we didn't see anyone at the nurses' station the whole time we were there. So my husband and I went out into the hallway and I told him I thought I should stay with Mom, that she shouldn't be left alone. He said that if we stayed, it would start a pattern that we couldn't reverse and we'd be there every night again. I agreed. We were both exhausted and had reached our limit.

I told the nurse that we were thinking of leaving, but I was concerned that Mom might try to get out of bed. He said he would give her a sleeping pill. I explained that if he did, she would be too groggy to do any physical therapy in the morning. So he said he would write on her chart to give her half of a pill. I told him I didn't think that would work either because she would wake up disoriented in the middle of the night and try to get out of bed. He said not to worry, he would check on her.

So we went back to Mom's room and I told her we were leaving. She said ok, and surprisingly didn't protest. We kissed her goodbye and promised to see her in the morning. Then we walked out. As we drove home, my husband and I talked about how guiltless she made us feel for leaving. It was the first time in over three months that one of us had not been with her.

At 6:30 the next morning, we got a phone call. A nurse at the rehab facility said, "Something has happened to your mother and they are taking her to the hospital. You need to go there right away."

Chapter Eleven: Journey's End

(They will leave the way they will leave.)

Following that alarming phone call from the nursing home, my husband and I quickly got dressed and rushed to the hospital. At this point, it had been five years since Mom's visit to the emergency room in Florida for her skin cancer; it had been three months since her sudden admittance to the emergency room in Ohio for her heart attack; and it had been exactly ten hours since we had left her at this latest rehab facility after her hip surgery.

I ran into the hospital emergency room yelling, "Do Not Resuscitate! Do Not Resuscitate!" but of course, it was too late. Mom had been found dead at the scene on the floor of the rehab facility and the emergency medical technicians had done cardiopulmonary resuscitation anyway. (The "Do Not Resuscitate" order I had signed was never seen or signed by the attending doctor, so the emergency medical technicians did not honor it.) We were led into a hospital room where Mom was lying on a gurney, an intubation tube sticking out of her mouth and an IV port still in her arm. Luckily, I think she had been dead for hours before they found her and did those awful things. But I was in shock. Why had she ended up like this? In those final hours, was she frightened? Or was she brave and determined to finally decide her own fate? I will never know, of course… but I prefer to imagine the latter.

I asked my husband to take his penknife and snip off a lock of Mom's hair, which I put in my pocket. Then I told the doctor we would stay and keep vigil until she went to the funeral home. The doctor encouraged us to go home and get some rest. It would be a while, he said.

That afternoon, I called the funeral home and was told they didn't have her. So I called the hospital. "Do you have her?" I asked.

"No," they said.

"Where is she?"

"We don't know," they said.

"You don't know?!" I said incredulously. "Well, who does?"

"Ma'am, you need to call the funeral home," came the answer, and they hung up.

So I called the funeral home again.

"This has never happened before," they said.

"Well, find her!" I said, on the verge of tears.

Three days later, they found Mom at the Sheriff's Department. She was having an autopsy.

"What?" I screamed. "WHY are they doing an autopsy?"

Evidently, in Ohio if it's been less than three weeks since someone has had surgery and then they die, an autopsy is required. Thank you very much, malpractice insurance.

When we finally got her, Mom's remains were cremated as she had wished, and the funeral home mailed her ashes to Florida via the U.S. Post Office so that our family could fly down and inter her next to Dad. (Since 9/11, if you carry cremated ashes onto an airplane they need to have a special clearance and to go through an airport security scanner, so I opted for what I thought was an easier route.) A few days before we were scheduled to travel, I called the cemetery in Florida to make sure Mom's ashes had arrived.

"Do you have them?" I asked.

"No, not yet," they said. (It had been over a week.)

I called the funeral home. "Did you send the ashes?" I asked.

"Yes," they said. "Last week."

"Well, the cemetery doesn't have them."

"We don't know what happened. We sent them," they replied.

"Then find them!" I said, feeling more than a little frantic.

Two days later, the funeral home called back.

"The post office can't find them. They're putting a trace on it." Are you kidding me??? First of all, shouldn't a person's ashes be sent by registered mail? And how ironic is it that Mom worked all those years for the U.S. Postal Service, and now they had managed to lose her ashes!

Luckily, the ashes were eventually located in another Florida city and forwarded to the cemetery just in time for her burial. For the interment, I brought along a white vase that had been sitting under the TV in Mom's apartment. After we arrived at the cemetery, the manager escorted me into his office and left me alone to place the ashes in the vase. On top of his desk sat a small, purple felt bag tied at the top with a skinny gold rope. Inside this bag was a clear plastic bag that contained Mom's ashes.

I sat down in the desk chair and took a deep breath. Then I pulled out the plastic bag and tried to lower it into the vase. The bag was bigger than I expected and the vase opening was too small. After grunting and pushing, I finally stood up and untied the bag and tried to squish it in. Some of the ashes escaped and squirted up into the air in a dark gray plume, which then rained ashes all over the desk. Horrified, I ran out to the mausoleum and got my husband to come back and help me. Together, we pried and squeezed the plastic bag into the vase until the contents fit inside. Then he left, and I was alone with Mom once more.

I sank back down into the chair and closed my eyes. Mom's final journey, our five-year odyssey together, was finally over. Every fiber in my being just wanted sit there and rest. But there was still one more thing to do. With a sigh, I stood up from the desk and reverently picked up the vase. Then I licked my fingers and blotted up all the fallen ashes that I could find - and rubbed them into my hair. (I certainly wasn't going to leave Mom in that room all by herself.)

Then I walked out and shut the door.

Epilogue

Six months after Mom's passing, most of her affairs had been taken care of. Her possessions were sorted and given away, or saved as keepsakes. A new resident moved into her apartment and immediately began redecorating. And the condominium association planted a red rose bush in Mom's honor, right below her balcony (red roses were her favorite flower.) I trim it every Spring and it's doing great.

Of course since then, there's been plenty to think about and plenty of time to think. I feel a sense of relief that I no longer need to worry about her. And I'm experiencing a new found freedom, I guess you could say, that I can finally schedule my day (and my life) without hesitation or fear of her suddenly changing my plans. Occasionally, I walk through a grocery store or stroll through a park and sadly remember the wonderful times we had, just Mom and me - some very, very sweet times.

I also reflect on the last three months of her life and the way she left - the pain, the humiliation and the countless medical interventions. We tried our best to help her, but was it enough? During that crucial time, I often reacted as her daughter rather than responding as her advocate. And unfortunately, there is also truth in the saying that "by not making a decision you are indeed making one."

In sharp contrast, about a year after Mom died, my husband's mother died also. She had cancer and was given a prognosis by her doctor of one month to live. I watched as her family rallied around her and celebrated her life before she passed. She was clear headed and dictated every last detail of her final days. Hospice came to her assisted living apartment, and on her last visit to her longtime doctor, she said, "We had a good run, didn't we?" She died in her own bed, with no invasive medical interventions and two of her children by her side.

I believe Mom, too, ultimately left on her own terms. She was done with the suffering. In fact, she was done with everything. And perhaps some good did come from it all. Perhaps that good is coming to you in the form of *Speaking Up For Mom*. I hope that you and your loved one will be encouraged to delve into its topics further, and to make your decisions wisely - because knowledge is power.

During what seems like a long time ago, when I was in the midst of Mom's care, I wrote a poem about her. I'm not sure if it does her justice, but it describes the mom that I knew:

My Mom…

Naive, yet daring

Gentle and kind

Yet a darker side (stubborn)

Afraid of anger, eager for love

Looking in the wrong places

Finding the wrong love

Wanting peace

Looking in the wrong places

Trusting me (sometimes)

But not trusting life

Loving the sunset

Yet never seeing the sun rise

Reluctantly aging

But aging gracefully

A kid in grandma's shoes

A reason to be alive

Not fear, but joy

For what was given

And hope that it was enough.

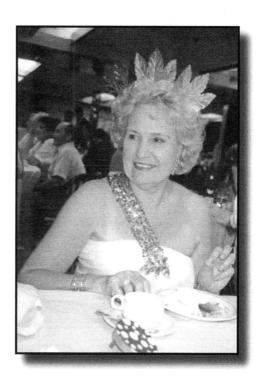

"The

Doctor

is In"

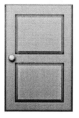

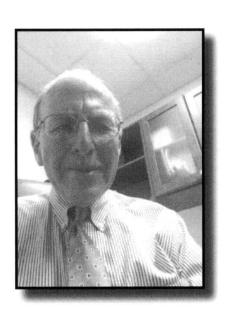

The Patient/Doctor Relationship

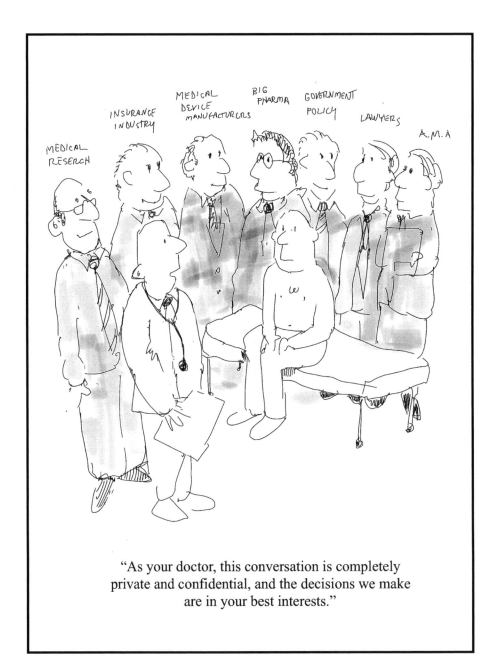

"As your doctor, this conversation is completely
private and confidential, and the decisions we make
are in your best interests."

Dr. Hanzelik On Improving the Patient Experience...

As a physician, what do you feel is the most important factor in a patient's health?

I think the most important factor is the patient's understanding of themselves and their active participation in protecting their own health. We each have a body and granted, there are certain weaknesses in our bodies. Yet, the human body is incredible. Think about how a baby is conceived, what it involves...two cells coming together. These cells are microscopic and you can't even see them and don't even realize that they're there. And yet they become that one little cell that embeds inside the uterus and now has all the understanding to create a heart, a brain, kidneys, an immune system. It's just phenomenal, and yet it's done so well so often, the vast majority of time we don't even think about it because it comes out just fine...but it is miraculous. Every human being is absolutely miraculous, as are all the other animals as well.

So we are given this human body and I think the most important thing for us to understand is that this body is a gift and we are the caretakers. No one else is going to take care of it for us. Doctors are just consultants, people who can help us to understand what is happening in our bodies. But the key to our health is the individual role that we each play.

What do you see as the biggest challenge facing physicians regarding patient care today?

I was reading recently that among all the industries in the U.S., the industry with the most regulations is health care. I think the reason for this is because medicine is so expensive and it's a big part of our country's gross national product - and it's becoming an increasingly larger part of it. So there are all these huge players who want to make money and influence the way medicine is practiced.

It's as if you are sitting in a room with your doctor, just the two of you, and you're having a conversation about the most intimate and most private aspects of your life. But also in that room, although you don't see them, are the medical association, the lawyers, the pharmaceutical companies, the national government, the society of doctors - all with their opinions. These entities have huge opinions on what constitutes good medicine, what is bad medicine, what a doctor should do or should not do. And the insurance companies now decide what medication you can use and they fight you on the cost of your prescription. So I think the biggest concern I have is regarding all these other people trying to squeeze into that little room and have their impact, and not really trusting the relationship that exists between the doctor and the patient.

From your perspective, what can a patient do to improve their experience and outcome in the medical arena?

The patient is the key. The arena is waiting there and at some point every person has to enter it. As a child, we are probably brought there against our will and we hate it, but we don't have much choice. When we become a young adult, I think it's important to start seeking out a doctor who we can trust and feel good about, who we can communicate with and who responds in a way that we perceive as very positive. We have to start working on that doctor-patient relationship early and the more we understand about ourselves, the easier the task of finding that physician will be.

I hear people making fun of others who look things up online, but I think the internet has tremendous potential. It has it's weaknesses, too. It can scare you to death when you read some of it because there's no control over who says what. But if you go to established medical websites, you can discover a lot of wonderful information about any problem. In my practice, I attract patients who are extremely interested in understanding their own situation. They bring books with them when they come to see me; they bring graphs they have made of their health; and they have lists of all these natural remedies that they take. They're incredible, and I love them for it and I totally support their engagement in their own health.

Some of my patients also reject standard medical procedures and there's certain things that I recommend to them that they still don't want to do. But I think that's fine and I work with them. Generally, we come to a very harmonious understanding because they understand that I'm on their side, I'm for them, I'm not representing any of those organizations I've mentioned before. I'm maintaining my independence and freedom, and my interest is the wellbeing of the patient. And they hear that and respect it, and they frequently ask me, "What would you do?" And I share my perspective. So I think people can play a very active role in finding a doctor in whom they can trust and communicate, be honest with and get really good advice.

I'd like to add that understanding ourselves, our bodies, our minds and our emotions is a challenging thing. Life is quick. Eighty years goes by very quickly. The more understanding we can have about what life is, how to enjoy it, even how to enjoy family, for instance, the better. I think family is an incredible creation, yet so often it goes berserk because of lack of consciousness and people can become mean and abusive and crazy, and it never needs to be that way. So, human beings need to work on themselves. Then they can take much better advantage of the health care arena.

In general, how can people avoid the scenario that happened in the story of Speaking Up For Mom?

Just as was illustrated in the story, I think a lot of people are in denial. They don't want to accept the fact that life has its limits, that we get old and that we do die at some point. It takes effort to really understand what life is and how to enjoy it and benefit from it. When we find health practitioners who we can really trust and communicate with, that's a real plus. But sometimes we need to work on ourselves. A lot of people have painful emotional experiences that ultimately affect their health.

Recently, I was seeing a patient who had many ailments but at the core of them was a great deal of anxiety. So I decided to get to the root of the problem rather than just address the symptoms. When I brought this idea up to the patient, she immediately began describing her painful childhood and some very traumatic experiences that had activated her internal stress system her whole life. Our stress system, if activated, will throw off all the health building systems of our body.

So the first thing I would suggest to anyone with internal stress is to find the ability to transcend those painful experiences that they've had as a child or an adult, and to engage the medical community to make it work for them. People need to recognize that the medical community doesn't automatically work for them. Just as doctors have so many regulations to abide by, patients have tremendous rules and regulations that they are under as well. For example, health insurance companies might say, "This treatment is covered, but this treatment isn't covered" or, "Yes, we will cover the cost of this medication but it will still cost you $900 after we've paid our share." It's very shocking for patients to hear things like this, but it's happening more and more.

So it's difficult for a patient to feel safe in the medical arena today, but it is doable. It takes some work - and I see many of my patients getting very skilled at it.

Dr. Hanzelik On Learning to Communicate With a Physician...

How do we develop skills for speaking more effectively with a doctor? What can we do to get better at this?

I think it's a very good question and I don't think there's an easy answer. In medical school, doctors don't learn a lot about communicating with patients. As individual physicians, we each have our own innate skill set but we really don't get intensive education on communication skills. So some doctors are good at communicating with patients and it comes naturally. They're listeners, they take in what people are saying, they make time for it. Other doctors may be very rushed, going from room to room, and they don't really have time to discuss anything. So it can be very intimidating and difficult to communicate with a doctor, particularly if the patient brings up questions about issues that the doctor has already decided upon. It can seem as if the patient is challenging what the doctor is saying. And if that challenge strays into areas that certain doctors do not respect very much - like dietary supplements or alternative treatments - then the doctor may develop an attitude very quickly about the patient.

So I think it's extremely important for the patient to communicate well with their physician. And if the patient needs someone to communicate for them, then that person must realize that to communicate well on behalf of their loved one, it takes some work on their part. Step number one is to do their homework and understand what is going on with the loved one. To do this, they need to have open communication with them, so that the loved one feels safe to share and the advocate can be in a position to help them.

The advocate, also needs to do their homework in terms of understanding their loved one's medical condition. If the doctor gives it a name, say, "Oh, the patient has cholecystitis," then there needs to be an understanding of what cholecystitis means. In this case, it's inflammation of the gall bladder which could be caused by gallstones or it could come from a blockage. The usual treatment is surgical, etc. So the advocate needs to prepare and think through some of these medical issues so that their questions to the doctor will make sense.

Now, I know it isn't necessarily easy for people to do this because they are often already upset that their loved one is in the hospital or they are worried about what could happen next. Or perhaps the advocate is busy and has their own family to deal with. But just taking a few minutes to research what is being said can make a huge difference in the communication with the doctor. And with our wonderfully smart cell phones we can look up anything on the internet very quickly and get an idea of what the doctor is talking about.

So, in the same way that doctors need to learn skills about how to communicate with their patients, patients and their advocates need to learn the skill of how to speak with the doctor, how to hold one's ground, how to be respectful and yet how to stand up for what one has to say. If you are communicating disrespect to the doctor, then that tends to undo the communication. So it's important to respect the doctor but that does not mean you need to agree with everything that person says, because you may have a different perspective and perhaps you can express it in a way that the doctor can hear it. I think this is an extremely important point and many doctors are prepared and ready for patient communication and are open to it. Therefore, I believe it's certainly something that people should work on and be prepared for and practice when they have the opportunity. And in the patient advocate role, these skills can play a very important part in the decision-making at any stage of a loved one's situation.

I've had experiences where if I question something a doctor says, they seem to take it personally. Is this experience unique?

It definitely happens, especially if the patient is interested in alternative treatments and starts mentioning dietary supplements, for example. The patient frequently gets strong reactions from the traditionally-trained doctor like, "That's completely worthless!" So it's definitely possible to get a strong reaction. But I think there are many doctors who won't respond in that way and who will respect the patient's feelings and input about their own plan of treatment.

When should a patient get a second opinion?

Personally, I feel that second opinions should be very common place, particularly if an invasive treatment is being considered. With surgery, for example, second opinions frequently make good sense depending on what is being proposed, for what reason, and of course, how urgent it is. Anytime there's a question or uncertainty in the patient's mind, a second opinion is a way to get another view of the situation and see if it matches the first view. However, if what the first doctor is proposing makes sense to the patient, if they feel very good about the doctor and the treatment is going well, then there's no need for a second opinion.

But if something significant is under consideration, it's very good to have another perspective. The more information the patient has can only be a benefit. The one drawback is financial. Sometimes health insurance will cover the second opinion, and sometimes it won't. But in general, I feel second opinions are very valuable and are worth the time and expense.

Should the patient tell their doctor when they are getting a second opinion?

It depends on the patient's relationship with the doctor. A lot of patients do tell their doctors. Often patients just say, "I'm going to see another doctor for a second opinion."

For instance, I had a patient recently who had injured her shoulder and her orthopedist would not strongly suggest that she have surgery. The patient wanted to resolve her shoulder issue quickly, so she and I discussed it and I supported the idea of her getting a second opinion - I even recommended the name of another orthopedist. Later, when I was talking to the first orthopedist, I mentioned to him that I had suggested that the patient see this other doctor. Hearing this from me, he seemed very positive about it. He said, "Oh that's fine. That's great. I think that will be good." And I believe his attention to that patient's care increased. The patient did see the other doctor but she felt more connected with the first, so she stayed with him. However, as a result of that second consultation, her care by the first doctor improved and it doesn't seem likely that she'll need surgery after all.

In general, how do doctors feel about their patients getting second opinions?

I think doctors accept it as a part of the game of practicing medicine. I'm sure there are doctors who wonder why it's necessary, but I think it's part of a patient's efforts to understand more about their own situation. And a doctor could use it as an opportunity to understand more about what the patient is feeling, such as, "Do you have any concerns that I am not addressing? Do you have any questions that I haven't answered? What can I do to help?" But at the same time, I think the doctor should be saying, "I think it's great to seek a second opinion because it will be useful for you. I support it fully."

Some patients seek out second opinions and don't tell their doctors - that happens a lot. I think the important thing to note about this is that the medical care system needs to be more user friendly for patients, so that the patient can navigate the system, can get what they need and can get good care. The issue isn't about how does the doctor feel. The issue is "what kind of care is the patient getting?"

Dr. Hanzelik On Treating the "Whole Patient"...

How common are adverse drug reactions in the elderly and what can patients, their caregivers or patient advocates do about it?

What we see developing in medicine today is an assumption that for every human ailment there is an unusual chemical substance which is the answer. We've all heard of the incredible side effects that occur with these substances. Just listen to any television commercial that advertises a medication and then cites its side effects. Yet, we seem to be in a state of denial about it, as if to say, "If I don't acknowledge the side effects, they won't happen."

Did you know that most of the medicines we take today block the normal functions of the body - for example, beta-blockers, channel blockers, ace inhibitors? These medications are created to block natural bodily responses and in doing so hopefully create side effects that might be beneficial. So that's why there are so many side effects. We're prescribing things that are at the same time alien to the human body and somewhat supportive of the human body.

Therefore, I think side effects and adverse reactions to medicines are extremely common. So patients or those who care for them need to be aware of the most likely side effects of any medication they take. The problem is that if you familiarize yourself with the side effects, you probably won't want to take the medicine or give it to your loved one! But it's a good idea to try to keep the use of medicines as minimal as possible; be aware (or ask) the loved one if the medications are helping or not; and know the most common side effects of the medication in case they present themselves.

One thing that patients or their advocates need to realize is that a patient can refuse any medical treatment at any time. Some patients are very proactive in deciding what treatments and/or medications they will accept. And some doctors resent this - but others appreciate it. Patients need a supportive environment to realize that they are in control. For instance, there's one blood pressure pill that I often prescribe who's most common side effect is an annoying dry cough. This may seem like a trivial side effect, but it's the main reason some people stop taking the medication. If that side effect occurs with my patient, I willingly suggest an alternative.

As I've said, I feel the human aspect of medicine is extremely important...helping people help themselves, helping people understand themselves, and helping people play a very active role in getting themselves well. Unfortunately, this aspect of medicine is not developing half as fast as I would like to see it happen! However, one thing that excites me is the current developments in alternative medicine.

Tell me about alternative medicine and why you think it's important.

Ever since my physician internship days, I've been looking for other ways of doing things, safer ways of practicing medicine. I've practiced wholistic medicine and now I practice integrative medicine. And one aspect of that is something called "functional medicine," where doctors are really doing things the way I like to see them done. Functional medicine looks at the functions of the body and tries to support them by recognizing that the body has an extraordinary potential to heal itself and get well. What the functional medicine physician tries to do is work with that innate healing capability rather than giving out these foreign substances to patients that block the functions of their bodies.

So, there are subtle differences between alternative, wholistic, functional and integrative medicine. If you go to the Functional Medicine Institute, they will tell you how functional medicine is different from everything else. If you go to an Integrative Medicine meeting, they will tell you how they are different. But in general, I think the words are used interchangeably and most patients don't know the difference between them. This whole alternative movement is really a revolution waiting to happen. Little aspects of it are getting accepted into the mainstream and people are slowly finding out about them and getting attracted to them, but it hasn't yet made the full leap into medical education and into the practice of traditional western medicine.

So, do you see alternative medicine offerings becoming more available or do you think that alternative and Western medicine will eventually merge?

I think these two sides of modern medicine, traditional and alternative, are coming together. More and more, alternative medicine is becoming mainstream. And traditional medicine will have to shift, because alternative medicine has a lot of truths in it that need to be recognized and accepted. So I'm optimistic that this transformation will happen. In fact, I feel that I've been a part of this shift for my whole career.

That's why I think communication with the patient is an aspect of medicine that cannot be neglected. I find it to be the most rewarding part for both the doctor and the patient, and it's in this arena where so much happens. These are the kinds of beings that we are - we can express ourselves really well and we can eventually understand ourselves. Actually, I think the essence of getting well is to understand ourselves, and medicine will eventually evolve to support that, although I think it will be a bumpy ride. But I think it will ultimately go in the right direction.

Dr. Mark Hyman, who is president of the Functional Medicine group, has done a lot of really good work. He was recently pursued by the Cleveland Clinic, which is a major traditional medical facility and very highly respected, to practice functional medicine there. He negotiated with them and they gave him an entire floor and a full staff, and now he's doing functional medicine for the Cleveland Clinic. I think a lot will come from that development, as traditional doctors see that traditional places can use an alternative healing method and benefit from it. So I think the way today's medicine is practiced is going to change. However, I've been at this for fifty years and it hasn't changed that much as of yet. So It's hard to say how long it will take.

Tell me more about your practice of integrative medicine. What kind of treatments does it include?

The first principle of integrative medicine is to look at the whole person when evaluating their health. The bio-psycho-social model taught in medical school is that when you treat a person there is a biological or physical aspect; a psychological or emotional aspect; and a social aspect (i.e., the patient's job, family, relationships.) All of these things can affect the person's health, and all of them need to be part of the consultation, because you don't really know which part is playing an important role for that particular patient. So that's principle number one of integrative medicine - treat the whole person.

Principle number two is to respect the extraordinary capacity of the body to take care of itself, to heal. It has a built-in healing mechanism, a built-in elimination mechanism, and an immune system. It has an extraordinary capacity. So a major role of the doctor is not so much to bypass that capacity, but to work with it. As a physician, how do I support the body? How do I help the patient function better so that their body can take care of its problems, rather than using strange chemicals (which is how I refer to pharmaceuticals) as the primary remedy?

Another area where integrative medicine differs from traditional Western medicine is the approach to treatment. We prefer natural remedies. We'll use pharmaceuticals when they are indicated and appropriate, but I think we use them less than traditional doctors do. In our office, we have a little natural pharmacy of our own, where we carry the products that we've had good results with, so people can get them here if they want. We also incorporate other schools of medicine. We've had an acupuncturist work with us and a massage therapist. We try to find other modalities that will help people get well, but are not as dangerous or toxic as traditional medical remedies.

How do you determine whether to use integrative medicine or Western medicine treatments with a patient?

That's not the way it works for me. I start out with a complete evaluation of the person, where I try and look at all the aspects affecting their health. Then I follow up with a second visit to go over the results of their tests and give my impression. And my impression comes from looking at the whole person, starting with the beginning of our encounter.

So, for instance, a major aspect of maintaining a person's health is their nutrition. Do they understand their nutritional needs? Do they have food allergies? Do they have digestive problems? Are they doing things that are going to help their body? We have a nutritionist in our office and a lot of our patients will see the nutritionist as well. So that's one area that is extremely important.

Stress is another health factor we focus on. I co-wrote a book called *The Inner Game of Stress*. Stress is recognized to affect every system in the body, and major health organizations have said data shows that 90% of all doctor visits include stress as a major factor for the visit. So it's important to recognize the detrimental affect of stress on our health. Yet, most doctors don't have an effective approach for dealing with stress. They may send the patient to a psychologist or start them on a tranquilizer, but those options are not what the patient really wants or needs. And frequently, doctors do not know how to deal with stress themselves.

Talk about medical specialities like geriatrics. Is it necessary to consider these when selecting a doctor for an elderly loved one?

I don't think it's necessary, but the value of seeing a geriatrician is up to the individual. Most internists (internal medicine physicians) are skilled at taking care of elderly people and I believe a geriatrician's approach wouldn't be very different. Sometimes, my elderly patients see me and they also see a geriatrician. Perhaps they get some ideas that are helpful. Whatever resource a patient can benefit from is fine with me.

Many health problems of the elderly are simple yet annoyingly persistent - like skin problems, digestive problems and high blood pressure. If these conditions get to be quite complicated, that's when specialists tend take over. So, at the level of the primary care doctor or the geriatrician, there's usually simple things that can be done that might help the patient. In some cases, it could be worth checking with a geriatrician, as they might know some useful tricks to improve the patient's situation.

However, taking care of the elderly is a major aspect of internal medicine. In fact, it's most of our practice. I have younger patients too (internists see patients age fifteen and above) and I like the diversity. And there are sub-specialists within internal medicine such as cardiologists, kidney specialists, endocrinologists, neurologists and dermatologists. A lot of times people will seek out these specialists for their care once they have a diagnosis, but I encourage them to keep seeing their primary care doctor in addition to the specialists.

Family care physicians, on the other hand, have a different training program from internists and most are trained to treat children as well as adults. I've always felt that a family care doctor is more of a general doctor, whereas internists are specifically trained to understand the internal workings of the body. Therefore, I've always seen internal medicine as a more in-depth understanding of what goes on in adults, and of course, all those sub-specialties I mentioned come from internal medicine. But there is a lot of overlap in the two areas of primary care, and some doctors in family care practice may be more knowledgable and capable than an internist. It really depends on the individual doctor. The most important factor is the attitude of the doctor - is he or she genuinely caring?

Are you hopeful that physicians, patients and their advocates can change the experience of medical care in the U.S.? If so, how?

The future of medicine is up in the air right now. Sometimes I hear, "Bring back the good old days of the country doc!" But I don't think the "Mom and Pop" medical practice is likely to happen again. Technology is tremendously influencing our society, not only in the way we live but also in the way we practice medicine. Advances in technology are not happening by normal addition, but exponentially. Normal addition might go 2,4,6,8,10,12,14 - whereas exponential multiplication goes 2, 4, 16, 256.

One example I give is about these little exercise trackers that people wear on their wrists. What these devices are capable of doing is expanding every day. Already you can do a full electrocardiogram or track your oxygen level by these things. So I think the growing role of technology in medicine is inevitable.

Medicine is going to change, but whether it will be entirely for the better requires a lot of individual effort to make sure the critical aspects of patient care do not get overrun. We've talked about the doctor's treatment room being packed with other forces. I'd put a few more people in there, too - the academics, the researchers and the technologists. They all sit in that room deciding what the doctor should do with the patient. A lot of doctors today don't even look at you during your appointment. They look at their machines the whole time they are working with you.

Granted, we want the most modern medicine, we want the best understanding, the best science - we don't want to compromise that. However, It needs to be balanced with the kindness and understanding of a real country doc. Technology will continue to move fast, but we have to contain it so that we maintain our humanity. The human aspect of medicine is often played down because people don't think it's important or relevant. However, I feel it's the most important part - the communication between the healer and the person. There is a lot that is communicated in that situation. I just don't think getting all your medicine from machines is going to do it.

What I am hoping for is a balance where doctors give their patients the best of both worlds. I think it is unlikely that individual doctors will do this on their own, however. It will probably have to be through physician groups which emphasize that type of care and give their doctors the freedom to practice heartfelt medicine. That's how I picture it. Right now, we have physician groups, but they are looking strictly to maximize profits by containing services. They're a financial model. A lot of the models out there right now are primarily financial rather than looking to enhance the overall quality of medical care. As an example, did you know there is a term for the vast amount of money spent on medical care in the last six months of a person's life? It is called "futile care."

If you feel the model of medicine that you practice is beneficial, why don't more doctors follow your example?

I think doctors are really open, and I'm hoping to do some work reaching out to doctors, and do some teaching to help doctors see the possibilities in practicing medicine. It's extremely challenging today, because all day long people come and share their problems, their worries, their fears, and your whole schedule is filled with...some have thirty patients a day. I have about twelve patients a day because I always schedule a lot of time with people. But there have been studies done that show the average time a doctor spends with their patient is 7 minutes. And doctors have this skill where they put one leg in the room and one leg out of the room, like they are ready to leave any second. So it really is a shift in attitude that is needed, to say, "The basic reason I practice medicine is simply to help people, and I'm not going to compromise that. When the insurance company says it's only going to pay me $15 for this service and I think its important for my patient, I will do it anyway."

Treatment

Vs.

Trauma

Dr. Hanzelik On the Trauma of Being Admitted to a Hospital...

Why is our medical system often such a frightening prospect for the elderly?

It's frightening for everybody. They have knives. They want to cut you. They have poisons that they want to feed you. They want to take you away from your family and lock you up in a room where nobody really cares about you. So it's a dangerous environment and the more we can stay out of it the better. It could be much more friendly and cooperative and kind and understanding, but it does not seem to be moving in that direction.

Right now, the big thing in medicine is technology, and I don't think technology is especially supportive of patient care and communication. So medicine keeps going through a transition, but not in the right direction in my opinion. I think the human aspect really needs a lot of development and it's currently being ignored.

Isn't it true that when we go into the medical system or a hospital, there's a sense of giving up control of perhaps the one thing we think we have control over - our bodies?

Yes, we're so private about our bodies. This is something that we really look at as "this is my private area." And in the hospital you lose that immediately. They tell you to take off your clothes. You no longer can just go to the bathroom when you need to. If you do need to, you might have to do it in the bed and they give you a little tray to use. So it's shocking in a lot of ways to discover this loss of choice and loss of freedom, and to discover that these areas which have been so private one's whole life are suddenly open to people who are strangers. And some of these strangers might communicate really well with the patient, and some might come across as brusk and rushed and irritable. And unfortunately, that second attitude is what comes across sometimes.

It seems like medical crises often occur at night or out of the blue. Is this true?

This depends mostly on the person's medical condition and how stable they are initially. Medical crises are more noticeable at night because the incident is scarier and there's more of a helpless feeling. For instance, heart attacks can occur at any time. However, during the day if a person has a little chest pain they can call their doctor and they have access to resources. At night, it's much more terrifying. The person either has to call the paramedics or do nothing. So I don't know if these situations necessarily happen more at night, but there are certain emergencies in medicine that can happen abruptly and suddenly, and when they hit it's an overwhelming and huge event. Usually, however, these issues have been developing gradually and silently for years before they actually happen.

How does this relate to the story in Speaking Up For Mom and what does the story mean to you?

I've been thinking about that question and it means a lot to me because of my experience. I see patients several days a week and I see a lot of elderly patients. And I see them when they are being hospitalized and when they are being informed that they need to be hospitalized. And I realize that as soon as the decision is made to hospitalize someone, the person is faced with a barrage of decisions that come very quickly and may be decided without even consulting the patient or their advocate. However, of all the decisions that a patient has to deal with, the first question needs to be, *"Should* I be hospitalized?"

If the answer is yes, then next comes a flood of questions regarding the hospitalization - such as,"What type of room should I have? Do I need to be in the Intensive Care Unit or do I need a regular room? Who will be my admitting doctor? Who will be the medical consultants on the case? What type of specialists do I need to see me? What type of tests do I need? What type of treatments? What are the side effects of the treatments? How will the treatments interact with the other treatments that I'm currently getting?" With all of these decisions to be made, the patient's doctor will have a strong position about what to recommend, so it really helps to have someone speaking up for the patient and offering them some support.

This is because these decisions are very scary and they have certain dangers associated with them - taking a particular medication can have serious side effects or having surgery can always have serious repercussions. So when someone is hospitalized, it's important to have a person who can assist the patient in speaking up, so the patient can contribute and participate. And if the patient can find a doctor who will make this process easier for them, who wants to hear what the patient has to say, who wants to know what their thoughts are on their own health, and instead of presenting just one choice to the patient, he or she presents three or four choices so the patient can participate in deciding what is best for them, that physician is a wonderful asset.

And supporting the decision-making and communication needs of an elderly patient - someone we love and care about who is in the hospital - and facilitating that communication, is extremely important. With the changes that are occurring in medicine, and potentially in health insurance coverage, there's so much uncertainty for people in an area that needs to be very stable and sensible and kind. So that's why I feel *Speaking Up For Mom* is so important, because this is an area where what the patient's advocate has to say plays a very important role in what is decided, and by listening to the patient and hearing what they want, cooperating with them, facilitating the communication with the doctor, all of these things will greatly enhance the likelihood of a very good outcome from a hospitalization.

What is the primary care physician's role when a patient enters the Emergency Room or hospital?

Let's be honest, doctors are maxed out. If a patient or the patient's advocate wants their primary care doctor to follow up with them in the hospital, they need to take the first step and keep after the physician. These days most hospitals use hospitalists, that is, doctors who only take care of patients in the hospital. Admittedly, this is a setback for the patient because the patient loses the supervision of a doctor who knows them well. For my patients, I try to stay in touch at least by phone, guiding the patient and offering support.

Something to note though...patients often choose to go to the emergency room (ER) when they have a medical problem rather than go to a private physician. However, ER facilities can only provide care for a limited time and are very expensive, often to the extreme. ERs are best called upon when it's necessary to rapidly diagnose unusual, sudden conditions and quickly begin treating them. Such situations tend to lend themselves to a lot of body scans in order for physicians to cover all their bases.

In the story of *Speaking Up For Mom*, we read how the mother, whom had clearly been traumatized by her previous medical interventions, began to depend on denial as a coping mechanism when she experienced new medical symptoms. What was needed in that situation was an open, friendly relationship with her primary care doctor. Unfortunately, she never found this relationship in a doctor. In fact, she never wanted to see a doctor again! She even felt safer going to an emergency room when her facial lesion appeared, even though the ER had very little help to offer. This illustrates that the primary care physician needs to be the first "port of call," and the patient needs to feel confident that their doctor is on their side and he or she will do whatever it takes to help them get well. I'll admit it's challenging to locate a doctor who you can truly trust to guide you and protect you in the medical care system. But these doctors do exist and are important to find.

Can the primary care doctor confer with the hospitalist to discuss treatment options for the patient?

Yes, the primary care physician can phone the hospitalist, which I do quite frequently. When I hear that one of my patients has gone to the hospital, I generally first try to speak to the patient in the emergency room. I let them know that I'm available and that they can call me if they have any issues at the hospital. I also try to speak with the hospitalist and establish a communication. Unfortunately, the communication is not ideal. There is one hospitalist who will text me most days about how my patient is doing, so that works out the best. At least, I have a sense of what's happening. Yet, it requires a lot of effort on the part of both of us. I have access to patient hospital records online and I can go through those records and open them up and see what a patient's lab results are, etc. But it takes a lot of time and doctors are busy people.

Can a primary care physician write orders when their patient is in the hospital, and perhaps override the hospitalist's orders?

I know of a hospitalist who routinely makes rounds from 1 to 3 a.m. So I wrote an order for one of my patients in his hospital that said: "Do not disturb this patient from 10 p.m to 7 a.m. Patient needs sleep. This includes doctor visits and vital signs." It helped. But primary care physicians have been somewhat pushed out of hospitals in recent years. I was the primary care doctor taking care of all my patients that were in the hospital until about two years ago. With hospitalists so prevalent, most primary care physicians are seeing patients in the hospital less and less, and allowing the hospitalists to provide the hospital care. And the primary care doctor and hospitalist can't both see the patient because health insurance won't pay for both.

So, I can choose if I want to take care of my own patient in the hospital. However, if I don't see patients in a particular hospital for a while, then the hospital tells me that I can't see patients there any more until I get approved because I'm "out of practice." Basically, it's a complicated situation. So, yes, the primary care physician can have influence on the patient's hospital care, but for most situations cannot write orders in the way that the hospitalist can.

Do you agree with the statement, "Our health care system is not really set up to serve people over 80 years of age?" Why or why not?

The challenges that people over 80 years of age face are serious medical issues. Of course, there's a wide variation. Some people are healthy into their 90's and some people are really sick in their 70's. But we have to recognize that old age has its unique features. It's a multi-faceted weakening of the body, and there's always the looming possibility of dying in the process of a medical procedure. So what we can achieve medically is limited.

People have a kind of fantasized view of surgery. "Oh, surgery...they'll just go in and remove my pain and I'll be back to normal." But you've got to realize that the tool that is being used in surgery is often a knife. When you think of your body, what can you accomplish with a knife? It's limited and it's painful. And yet, surgeons do open heart surgery on people who are 85 years old!

As I've said, people come to me for medical clearance for surgery and my first question to them is, should they have the operation? I've convinced a lot of my patients that they are better off without an operation. And by and large, it's worked out really well. Frequently, they do fine without surgery and their symptoms disappear and don't come back.

I'm an integrative doctor so I'm always looking for natural remedies that can help people. And I think there are lots of things that can help. But with the elderly, we're working against death, so a doctor can do everything that they can, but there's still a force that is taking the person down. So it's a delicate path to walk. But I have several patients in their 90's and they're amazing. Some of them are really vibrant and energetic and doing well.

Dr. Hanzelik On Choosing the Best Treatment Options...

Explain your definition of invasive versus non-invasive medical procedures. Does it change with the situation?

Invasive procedures are ones that go deeper into the body. If you put a cream on your skin, for instance, that's not invasive, it's very superficial. But if you give an injection, that's a little more invasive. If you actually cut into the body and remove something, that's a little more invasive. If you put the person to sleep so that they're under full anesthesia and then you open up a body chamber, that's maximally invasive. So it's kind of logical that the level of invasiveness means how deep you are going into the body for that particular procedure.

Is age a determining factor in whether surgeries and other invasive procedures should be pursued?

Age isn't as much of a factor in determining the line of treatment as is the person's physical condition. I'll give you an example. I had a patient who was eighty-six years old and he had seen an orthopedist and the orthopedist recommended that he have major back surgery. I was doing the pre-op clearance, that is, evaluating him to see if he was medically cleared for surgery. As I examined him, I found a number of major issues with his health. His heart rhythm was irregular, and when I checked, he was in atrial fibrillation - an abnormal rhythm of the heart. Then I checked his lungs and he had evidence of pretty advanced cardio pulmonary disease (COPD), which is like emphysema. Plus his blood pressure was very high, 200/130.

So he had a lot going on medically, and I told him I could not approve him for surgery. But he wanted to proceed with it because he had been told that he needed the surgery and he really wanted to have it. So he went to a cardiologist and a lung specialist, and eventually they both cleared him for the surgery. When I finally got the report on this patient, I found out that he had had excessive bleeding, kidney failure requiring dialysis and sepsis. He did not survive the surgery. The warning signs were loud and clear, but he found doctors who would ignore them.

So I'm constantly advising people not to have surgery who are scheduled to have it. I call it balancing the pros and cons. If you're trying to make a decision, write down all the good things that can come from that decision and all of the potentially bad things. Then you can look at the list and usually it's pretty obvious what decision to make. There are patients in their 90's who have had operations that they have benefitted from and that were valuable for them, and there are patients in their 40's who have had serious complications and very serious problems from surgery. So definitely age is a factor, but it's not the key to the decision - it's more about the patient's condition, what operation is being proposed, how likely they are to benefit from it, and how likely they are to have complications afterward.

Post-op is the amount of time it takes to recover from surgery - to get up on one's feet, to get mobile and to establish adequate food intake. If there are surgical wounds, they need to be kept clean and dry and well protected so that they don't get infected. There's a lot of issues in the post-op period and the more health concerns brought into it from the pre-op period, the more difficult it is to recover and get well.

Here's a very common situation...An elderly person falls and breaks their hip, perhaps late at night, and then is taken to the hospital. The surgeon is very strongly oriented toward doing the operation and wants to do it early the next morning because he or she knows that if they don't operate and fix the hip, the person will never walk again. But the patient and/or their advocate needs to understand the pros and cons of the choice to operate and to think them through, and then come to a decision with the doctor.

The patient could have the surgery, that's one option, but it means anesthesia, post-operative pain and physical therapy with painful legs. It's going to be quite a difficult recovery. But if the patient doesn't have the surgery, they will have pain from the fracture, they will be bedridden and completely immobilized and will probably die. Either way, the patient will probably die. So it's a very difficult situation. Some people opt not to have the surgery, but I'd say the majority of people opt to do it because it's such a pressure situation for the patient or their advocate - the surgeon really wants to do it.

I've advised patients in this scenario many times, and in many cases, I've felt there were good results from having the surgery. The patients become functional and have some life left because they had the operation. On the other hand, if a patient's overall health is very poor and their likelihood of recovering is very small or they just don't want the surgery, then yes, there are situations where it's obvious the person is just too ill to go ahead. There are then two choices and neither one is very appealing.

I have a patient who is ninety-five and who had the hip surgery, but she never did the physical therapy that was required, so she never started walking. I kept urging her, "Do the physical therapy. Do the physical therapy." But she never did. It's now been a couple of years since her surgery and she's been on total bed rest for those two years.

The story in *Speaking Up For Mom* is another example. Such a sad tale and yet, one that is happening thousands of times throughout our country every day. It's true that if surgery is not done for a broken hip the person will not be able to walk and often will die soon. But we have to ask ourselves if the person can survive the surgery and with what quality of life. The mother in this story needed a serious hospice evaluation when her daughter first brought it up, and then again when the nurse mentioned it in the rehab facility. Hospice shifts the focus from invasive to non-invasive, from intervention to comfort, from being lost and confused in the hospital to having time to say goodbye to the people you love. This mother and her daughter needed someone experienced in the medical arena to help them navigate this dangerous hospital terrain. Sometimes a doctor or a nurse will assume that role, but often the patient's advocate is left on their own to face those heart-wrenching decisions.

Suppose the hospitalist doesn't want to listen to the patient or the patient's advocate regarding their preferences for treatment, what would you say to that?

Talk with your patient, the loved one, if they are capable of having a conversation. Decide together how serious you want to be about pursuing an alternative situation. Most hospitals have a bioethics committee and will allow you to present an ethical issue to them, such as when you feel the patient wants a particular option and it is not being offered. Or you can bring it to a formal review at the hospital if you feel the treatment is strongly going against what the patient wants. If you are the legal health care proxy (*see "Dr. Hanzelik On Having a Voice In One's Medical Care"*) and the patient can't speak for themselves, you can initiate something along those lines on your own. In other words, you do have recourse.

But first you have to decide if the situation is worth fighting for. Is the patient going to die very soon, and if so, is it worth the fight? If it is, speak to your loved one's doctor and say, "We cannot accept this situation. We really feel something needs to be done. What are our options?" The doctor will communicate some options to you and you can see if that satisfies the situation. Or you can call on hospice to work with the patient. Or speak with the bioethics person at the hospital. There are a lot of ways to speak up for the patient because hospitals are legal facilities licensed by the state and therefore sensitive to criticism.

If your loved one is in the hospital and you feel you just cannot work with the attending physician, what can you do?

You can request to have a different attending physician. You can say, "It's just not working out. We'd like to switch to a different doctor." However, then you have to find a doctor who is willing to take on the situation under those circumstances. The hospital might help you. A lot of hospitals have a staff member available to deal with patient issues that arise. So if you can identify someone like that, you can say, "It's just not working out with this doctor. Can we get another doctor?" and they can definitely arrange it for you.

What is the role of the hospital social worker? To be a patient advocate or to advocate more for the hospital than for the patient?

The hospital social worker definitely works for the hospital, but some of them are also patient advocates. However, some hospitals have a separate person on staff as a patient advocate to take on that role. So if you feel it is needed, check with the hospital staff to locate the right person.

What are your thoughts about those who are AMA (Against Medical Advice) patients?

This is a legal situation. It usually occurs in the emergency room or the hospital where the doctor is recommending something and the patient chooses to leave the situation. The doctor wants to make it clear that he is not telling the patient to leave, that the patient is leaving against his medical advice. So the doctor says they can leave, but they will need to sign this recognition that they are choosing to leave against medical advice. Some patients refuse to sign it, and they can't be forced to do it. It's basically the doctor protecting himself, saying, "I told the patient they should stay, but they insisted on leaving and what happens afterward isn't my fault."

Can the person who is AMA go back to the same facility or doctor, if needed?

Yes, they can usually go back. I've heard that sometimes insurance companies won't pay for a person's treatment if they go against medical advice, but I don't really think that's true. I believe it's just a threatening tactic, trying to manipulate the patient. Or it may be the doctor trying to protect himself by saying, "Ok, you're choosing to go out of the facility but be clear that I'm not telling you to do that." Doctors can be extremely intimidating, and a lot of doctors feel the patient shouldn't say squeak. Do you realize that when a doctor writes down what a patient is supposed to do, it's called the patient's "orders"? It's a military model. The doctor issues the orders and the nurses have to carry them out. So this whole attitude about medical care needs to shift - and it's doing so very slowly.

I yelled at a nurse once during Mom's first hospital stay, but I sought her out later and apologized. I was so frazzled seeing them perform a procedure that caused Mom pain, it just sent me over the edge. However, they did stop the procedure.

It's good when there's someone with the loved one who cares that that person is suffering. The question is, can life be extended or can pain be diminished? Sometimes we approach these two things as if they are opposites. Perhaps to extend life does mean taking on more pain and more suffering, but perhaps it does not. So you want to have balance in your decision-making such that you are aware of what's too much, and what's not too much. Thus, the patient or their legal health care proxy may be willing to consent to one treatment or procedure, but not willing to consent to a different treatment or procedure. Again, it's important that the patient feels protected and that someone is on their side.

I do a lot of consultations where I understand the procedure that the hospitalist wants to undertake and I explain the procedure to my patient. When the patient fully understands it, then they are in a position to say, "That will be ok," or "No, I don't want that." However, for a patient to be able to say, "No, I don't want that," their understanding of the procedure is required. Doctors need a patient's approval (or the health care proxy's approval if there is a legal arrangement) to do a procedure. The doctor can't just do a procedure without patient approval. So in the story of *Speaking Up For Mom*, for instance, you gave initial approval for those procedures which you ultimately objected to and demanded that they stop. But you did give the initial approval.

(Yes, this is true.)

Dr. Hanzelik On the Crucial Role of Patient Rehabilitation...

Unlike a younger person who goes to the hospital for an operation and then comes out and recovers fine; for the elderly, isn't the hospital so dangerous that they may not come out at all or they may come out with only half the functionality they had before?

I see a tremendous challenge when an elderly patient enters a hospital. No patient wants to, of course, but sometimes it's necessary. Yet, it's extremely threatening for an elderly person. It's threatening to a child, too. It's threatening to everybody. But for an elderly person, it's a disruption to the entire stability in their life.

Just like a child, the elderly patient really needs someone to support them when they are in the hospital - to protect and communicate for them. If left to themselves, these patients are going to feel very insecure in the hospital and that feeling itself is very disconcerting. These patients are in a new environment, with new people, in an unfamiliar situation and there's all these rules. The person probably has an IV (intravenous medication) running and tubes coming out of different orifices of their body. It's not a fun situation.

I used to call an elderly person's reaction to this situation "the senior dwindles," meaning that from just being hospitalized, the elderly patient's health can start to get worse. And yes, it's true, that elderly people go into the hospital and sometimes they don't come out. That definitely happens.

Why are elderly persons often recommended for rehabilitation after a hospital stay?

As I just mentioned, hospitalization is often a devastating experience for the elderly. It's just a natural fact of life that we are mortal and we don't live forever. And the aging process is built into our biological system. So this means that at some point we are going to need to enter the health care arena, and that arena has some very nice and wonderful aspects to it, but it also has its risks and dangers - and sometimes people end up getting hurt. Elderly people are already frail and gently getting by, and then the hospital removes their freedom, their familiarity, their comfort, even their mobility.

There were studies done recently which showed that the third most likely cause of death and disability in the U.S. after heart disease and cancer is something called "iatrogenics." Iatros is a Greek word that means "we did it". In other words, the medical problem was created by the medical treatment itself. There's even a fifteen-hundred page textbook on the subject that lays out all the potential complications of surgery, pharmaceuticals and radiation - treatments being used in a hospital. In fact, when a person is admitted to a hospital they are subject to all sorts of unusual infections that they normally might not get. And then there is the incidence of hospital delirium, a hospital phenomenon which is usually due to the disorienting impact of the hospital environment. So why do patients often end up in a hospital in the first place? Many times, it's due to a physician's fear of lawsuits and the desire to protect themselves. But actually, we should only use hospitals if we really need them, as they are places that can be super dangerous.

Once in the hospital, a patient can benefit from their hospitalist writing orders to get them out of bed quickly and add physical therapy to their daily regimen to help maintain or regain their strength. And as soon as the patient is able, if more therapy is needed, a doctor's order for rehab means the patient can now be moved to a somewhat safer environment outside the hospital for further recuperation. To the patient or the patient's advocate, it may sound like the doctor is ordering them to "transfer to a rehab facility," and it may sound very intimidating. But it's always the patient's or health care proxy's choice to refuse admittance to a rehab facility and to try rehab at home.

Do rehab facilities really work for the elderly?

I think rehab facilities have the potential to work for the elderly but they frequently don't - sometimes it's because the facility is not especially good and patients don't get the kind of attention they need. Hospitals don't make enough income on patients who are just doing rehab and don't need other medical procedures, so these patients are often sent to rehab facilities because hospitals don't want to keep them. Thus, patients end up in a lesser facility that has less equipment and a less skilled staff (although, this really depends on the facility.) Plus, elderly patients are often weak, unmotivated and depressed, which is frustrating for the rehab staff who has to work with them, because the patient's progress is not that great. Therefore, it's very easy to neglect elderly patients - and when that takes place, then bad things happen. So all these forces work against an elderly person's recovery. And most elderly patients do not like rehab facilities and want to get out. But rehab itself is essential for getting well. Patients need to get back on their feet, get their appetite back, start taking care of themselves again, and regain their brain function.

Can dementia patients get adequate care in a hospital or a rehab facility? If so, what does it take?

I definitely think dementia patients can get well in a hospital, but they are much better off if someone like the health care proxy or a family member is with them at all times, to protect them and make things go easier for them. The person who knows the patient best needs to explain to the hospital staff, "Accommodations need to be made because this patient has dementia symptoms. Here are the things that the patient can talk about and these are the things that they really can't."

In general, the hospital staff is very busy and overwhelmed so someone who is demented is very difficult to handle. The nurses want to be sensitive and caring, but it depends on what kind of dementia the patient has. If the patient is agitated and screaming, the nurses may want to move them somewhere else and may tend to resort to medications to slow down the patient so they can't carry on too much. It's not a good situation.

Yes, often in medical facilities, you can feel the stress among the staff...

That is a very important factor in the quality of patient care because medical facilities are difficult places in which to work and they are usually understaffed. There's more work than there are people to do it. I have a good friend who's a nurse at a hospital here in Los Angeles, and she's constantly exhausted. She feels such a challenge everyday trying to keep up with the demands of her patients. So nurses do care and they want to do a good job, but it's difficult because of the increasing demands of the job and the lack of staffing.

I realize that the patient, the patient's advocate and the medical staff are all part of the same team, wanting to do what is best for the patient. However, if the advocate is stressed, worried and/or functioning on lack of sleep and yet needs to communicate effectively, isn't that quite a challenge?

I know how difficult it can be, and yet a lot rides on it. This is where the understanding comes in - that to do this task well of being an advocate takes responsibility and takes effort. Some people get hysterical and emotional and create a scene at the hospital. That really doesn't go over well.

Dr. Hanzelik On the Challenges of Caregiving...

What would you like to say to today's caregiver?

People are generally not ready to take on the role of caregiver. It's not easy to take care of an elderly person and sometimes there are already conflicts in the family - one person feeling, "Why am I the only one taking care of him or her? Why aren't my brother, my sister, our cousins helping?" So it's a very challenging role, particularly if a little bit of dementia is added to the situation and the patient is not totally cooperative.

It can be extremely difficult to work with a person who has dementia because you are used to that person "being there." When a person's brain is not working, it's as if they are not really there and you can't share things with them. I've seen families deal with this situation in many different ways. Sometimes, the family just can't manage the loved one at home. Perhaps they have to work or they have children at home, and they can't provide the services that are needed. At those times, it does require finding the right type of facility. In other cases, people are able manage their loved one at home. Certainly, most patients prefer to die at home. At least, that's their preference. However, it often doesn't happen that way unless the family really prepares ahead for the possibility.

In the story of *Speaking Up For Mom*, for instance, it was clear that the mother was developing dementia a few years before she died, and after her hospitalizations this became a major aspect of what was going on with her medically. Her brain was not functioning as well as it used to, and she was at the point where she couldn't live by herself. So if I had been her doctor at that time, I would have taken the opportunity to sit down and communicate with her and her loved ones, to understand what was going on, to share the options that I saw, and to put them in touch with resources that could be helpful. What actually happened in the story developed over a couple of years' time; it wasn't just in the last three months of the mother's life. So a lot of things could have gone differently if the family had had the support they needed and could have thought through their decisions more carefully, rather than constantly guessing what was the right thing to do under the pressure of a medical emergency.

There's one other point I'd like to make. Sometimes it does seem like the health of the person we are caring for plateaus and then plummets, plateaus and then plummets again. This is a sign that things are not going well. When things are going well, the person feels better, then plateaus, then feels better, then plateaus. Occasionally, a patient does have a minor plummet but the trajectory is that the patient is feeling better. Diet, among other non-medical factors, can often play a role in this trajectory. Nutrition is not a popular subject with most doctors but it's important to recovery.

What are the challenges when an elderly person needs to downsize their lifestyle?

We have these different chapters in our lives, and each of these chapters has its challenges. Childhood has its challenges, puberty, the 20's, 30's and 40's. And in the 70's, 80's and 90's, there are unique challenges of that time period, i.e., medical issues and downsizing living arrangements. The more prepared we can be, the more openly we can look at these challenges and honestly communicate about them, the more we will find our resources and listen to them and benefit from them, and the more likely things will go very smoothly.

Downsizing is extremely difficult for elderly people because they are often entrenched in their homes. They may have occupied their houses or apartments for forty years or more! Regardless of how long they've lived there, most are very uncomfortable with moving. Change in general is difficult for them - but especially so when it involves disrupting one's entire life and moving everything they own from one place to another. Then there's the issue of entering a new community where their friends are not there; the people they know casually are not there; all the comfortable things in their life are not there. It's very disorienting. And if the person has a little bit of dementia. that adds to the challenge - and in this new situation, the person will most likely appear even more demented.

I think we can admit that none of us are really prepared for getting old and dying. These are shocking aspects to our lives that we are not prepared for. We fight them, we resist them, we don't believe in them. . .I feel the same way. The thought of moving out of my house, and all of the things that our family has accumulated over the years - it's overwhelming to think about! So the conversation about end-of-life care can really help people start to communicate their anxieties about this and develop the skills needed to handle these kinds of transitions.

As to where someone in this situation should move, there are various alternatives. If the person has gotten to a point where they can no longer live by themselves and it's possible to be in the home of an adult child or relative, for example (if it works for the family,) I think that's a very good possibility. My wife and I had that arrangement for my wife's father. It was definitely nice for him and for us, too. However, when things got to a point where it became too much for us to care for him, he was moved to an assisted living facility where he lived for several months before he died. We were happy with the care he received there and it seemed to work for him. Yet, every situation is different and finding the best solution for a loved one can be very challenging.

In some localities, there are services available to help people find appropriate living situations for their elderly loved ones. These people know all the local facilities and can help connect the family with what is available. However, it's never a simple decision. Sometimes people try to make caregiving work at home by hiring someone to come into the home on a regular basis. If they happen to connect with a really good person, that person can become an incredible help. The hired caretaker might do the loved one's bath or provide their food or change the diapers. This can make it much easier to keep the loved one at home. However, this arrangement is fairly expensive and it's not covered by health insurance or Medicare. So there are lots of different options available but you have to find what works for you.

I've heard that a doctor, at the behest a patient's family, might talk to the patient about their future living arrangements or the need to stop driving, perhaps saying something like, "Your present living arrangement is not going to work for you long term and you need to decide what to do and where to live in the future," or "Perhaps you should consider no longer driving for your own safety."

Yes, definitely the primary care physician or geriatrician can facilitate these sensitive communications. I've been asked to talk to patients about not driving a car. Sometimes the doctor notifies the DMV that the person needs testing for their ability to drive. The doctor can also discuss the suitability of living situations. Many families recognize what is happening and start making their own plans. But families who want the support of their doctor should bring their concerns to the doctor and she/he will address them in their own way.

A Voice

Not

A Victim

Dr. Hanzelik On Having a Voice In One's Medical Care...

What is a "health care proxy" and why do we need one?

The "Durable Power of Attorney for Health Care" is a legal document wherein you name the person or persons who you trust to make health care decisions for you - if for any reason you are not capable of making those decisions for yourself. It's more than a piece of paper. The person(s) you choose in this document needs to be able to connect with you and make sure that they understand your approach to life and the kind of medical decisions that you would want to be made. So you need to choose a person with whom you have confidence and can have an open conversation and who is willing to communicate for you.

The role of this person, sometimes called a "health care proxy," is not one of being the original decision maker, but to implement what your choices would be in those circumstances if you could convey them. And having a health care proxy is something that really applies to all of us. We may not like it, but we don't automatically live to age ninety and then die. People die as children, as teenagers, in their 20's, 30's and 40's. So serious illness and death can occur at any point in life. Therefore, the health care agent or proxy is an important bridge between the patient and the medical care system.

Their main role is to understand what the patient wants and to help them get it. The proxy needs to know how to listen and also how to speak up. And they need to encourage the patient to talk about their perspective, i.e., what do you want from your care? What are your fears? What are your hopes? What are you feeling in your body?

If I am asked to be someone's health care proxy, what do I need to do?

If someone asks you to be their health care proxy, I think you should say, "Is there anything that you would like me to know now, that relates to your health or your approach to your end-of-life care plans, in case there is a medical emergency? Because the more I understand, the more I will be able to help you if anything happens."

This "end-of-life care" discussion is a relevant way of asking, "If you were to become really sick what do you want?" And in that conversation the person might have to ask themselves, for example, "If my brain was not functioning or I lost a lot of brain function, or if my condition was incurable and I was not going to survive it, would I want my life prolonged as much as possible? Or would I want some medical care, but there are certain treatments that I wouldn't want? Or would I just want 'comfort care'?"

What we are saying is to be prepared, make that effort, sit down and talk with your loved one and say, "For me to do this job well, the more I understand about your health the better. So if anything is going on, it would be helpful for me to know." The loved one may actually be grateful to have someone to communicate with. In many situations, I think they will be. And in this conversation, the health care proxy doesn't really need to make any recommendations to their loved one. The proxy is just there to take in what is being said, to listen, and to get an understanding of that person - which will help the health care proxy do his or her job if a medical emergency arises.

Also, it's best if the health care proxy does their homework, using reliable sites on the Internet like Medscape.com or MayoClinic.org, to gain a good understanding of the patient's conditions, so that they are prepared to discuss the patient with the patient's doctors. Amazing recoveries are possible if the patient is motivated to get well, the proxy understands his or her role and the doctor is committed to helping the patient recover.

Are there challenges to being a loved one's health care proxy?

The main challenge is really taking the time and having the communication skills to understand what the loved one feels is important in their life, what they want. It's often a difficult conversation to have because most people are reluctant to speak about dying or preparing for dying, and they often haven't thought it through. Some people are pretty comfortable with the subject, but most are reluctant to talk about it. So that's the main challenge for people who agree to sign the "Durable Power of Attorney For Health Care" as a health care proxy - to understand deeply what their loved one wants in case it is needed. One never knows exactly what situation they will be in, what medical emergency will be going on or whether the patient will be conscious or unconscious at that time the proxy is needed. It's all of a bit of a shock when it happens, so being prepared is the crucial issue.

Also, there can be obstacles. There's the whole aspect of denial. People do not like to acknowledge that they have medical problems. And there's a fear that their condition may be worse than they think it is. Or they imagine that they may be labeled with something that will be life-limiting (i.e., driving with a memory impairment.) So it's not an easy area in which to communicate. But if the health care proxy is coming from a place of caring, kindness and compassion, the loved one will eventually open up and share - and the safer the loved one feels, the more they will share. So creating a safe environment for that communication is extremely important.

Can previous relationship issues with the loved one affect the ability of the health care proxy to help?

Yes. If there is a lack of trust between the loved one and the health care proxy, this makes decision-making much more difficult. In order to make good decisions and to really understand what the loved one wants and what situations they would be satisfied with in their end-of-life care, it's important to build that trust. And it's often difficult to do because there may be a long history of uptightness, anxiety or fear about treading into such uncomfortable territory.

So it takes time...and the way to overcome these obstacles is to let love be at the forefront of the relationship. Convey that you are doing what you are doing because you care, and that you want your loved one to have the best possible experience because you love them. The more a person can hear this and start to trust it, the less any difficulties of the past will be an issue. I think it's extremely important to be able to listen and hear what the loved one is saying - and to repeat back to them what you *hear* them saying - so that they can tell you whether or not you are hearing them correctly, and whether they feel comfortable with your understanding.

However, it's a delicate dance, and sometimes the loved one can get angry or upset during this kind of conversation. Or they become incoherent because they have some dementia. That's definitely a major aspect of the challenge. And we need to understand that this whole experience of dependency is new for the person going through it. They're not usually prepared for dying or for being really sick and unable to take care of themselves. So there's this very real feeling of "I don't want to be a burden." It's quite common for people in such a situation to feel that and it makes it harder for them to be helped. I'm constantly advising my patients in those situations to allow others to take care of them. But people are concerned for their adult children or their spouses and don't want to give them a lot of worries and difficulties. So it's challenging.

If an "end-of-life" care conversation has not taken place and then a medical emergency arises, can't this be quite a challenge for the health care proxy?

Yes, that's true. The fact that we are mortal, that illness happens, that death happens - these things are not just possible, but guaranteed. And it's hard to talk about them. It's hard to bring up the subject, especially with people we love. But I think at some point in the future of medicine, having this discussion will be a natural thing, and we will be able to share about it and look at it honestly - perhaps even with some humor. And if a medical emergency is not looming over us, we will be able to plan ahead and feel confident that when something eventually does happen, we will know what to do. There will be a calm sense of, "I know what I am going to do. I know how to handle it - and I know how to use the medical care system." That last one is a big one. Certainly, being prepared to utilize the medical care system would have made a huge difference in the experience we read about in the story of *Speaking Up For Mom*.

If the health care proxy is having difficulty initiating this conversation, can the loved one's primary care physician help?

Typically, the conversation first begins among family members. Perhaps the health care proxy talks with their siblings or other adult family member(s) about what's going on with the loved one, and what can possibly happen next. Then the family decides to talk directly with the loved one and perhaps express, "We are worried about you. These things are happening…and we are considering different options," to see if the loved one will discuss it. From the proxy's meeting with family members and then with the patient themselves, hopefully some possible solutions get sorted out. At that point, after those conversations have taken place and the family has tried working with the loved one, it might be a good time to bring up the subject to the primary care physician.

Unfortunately, a lot of doctors want to play down their role in the conversation or make it about legalizing certain decisions, rather than really facilitating the conversation. A book called *The Conversation* by Dr. Angelo Volandes addresses how doctors can facilitate this end-of-life discussion with their patients, and this book can be very helpful to the physician. The doctor who wrote it is trying to train primary care doctors to become skilled at carrying out these conversations and to be willing to do so. He wants to create a revolution where the conversation about life-sustaining treatment is an automatic part of the relationship that doctors have with their patients, and that family members have with each other. So hopefully the topic will eventually be out in the open and it will be something that people will communicate about.

Does this conversation need to be updated now and again depending on changing circumstances (i.e., home care is no longer possible or dying at home is not feasible?)

Yes, the conversation is very dynamic and has to evolve as the situation evolves. Often the provisions of how the loved one's wishes will be carried out are somewhat vague at the outset, because the person and their proxy don't actually know what will be possible at the actual time those decisions are needed. That's why the spirit of cooperation between the loved one and the health care proxy and other family members is so important. And the person in the family who is providing most of the care and support to the loved one needs help, acknowledgment and appreciation from the other family members. As time passes, the more that the caregiver responsibility can be shared among the family members and perhaps new alternatives can be considered, the better for the patient, the caregiver and the proxy.

I've heard that if there are several family members involved with the loved one and one person is designated as the health care proxy, there are times when the proxy

may seem to "take over"and not want others to participate in the loved one's care or decision-making.

This is very much influenced by the ongoing relationships among all the potential players with each other. It can be very challenging to provide support to an elderly patient. The best scenario is when the health care proxy and the back up proxies and interested parties all work together and share the responsibilities of taking care of the loved one, so it can be as pleasant as possible for the supported person. However, everyone has their own way of doing things and the potential for conflict abounds. I say "be wise and steer clear." The chance to witness this stage of a loved one's life is a gift. It can enhance the lives of those involved. However, we can't change each other. I suggest focusing on doing our part as best we can and steering clear of conflicts.

Sometimes when a health care proxy is dealing with the patient's other family members, it's difficult. One person may be feeling that the patient does not want a lot of involved care and invasive procedures and that they just want comfort care. Another family member may be really terrified of that person dying and want everything possible to be done to save the patient. So this becomes a real conflict at a very difficult time if it hasn't been worked through previously. And it does happen where different members of a family with very different perspectives on what is important for the loved one can, unfortunately, get very angry with each other.

Another area that sometimes becomes an issue is money. The inheritance that the loved one is leaving behind becomes an issue and conflicts arise between members of the family even before the person has departed. There's a lot of potential conflict regarding how the money should be handled, and that can get in the way of just being present when the person is in the process of leaving. Sometimes people are even in a hurry for the person to pass. It's a situation that can bring out a lot of craziness in people.

Anything else you would like to say to today's health care proxies?

What was communicated in the story of *Speaking Up For Mom* is really a very common experience. Hospitals are not necessarily very patient-oriented. I like the title *Speaking Up For Mom* because indeed that's what it takes. It takes the health care proxies, the people who care, to speak up for their loved ones. They have to really defend the individual who enters the hospital.

In the book *Medical Nemesis* by Ivan Illich, he says, "Do not go into a hospital unless you have someone with you to protect you." I, as a doctor, have been in hospitals for many years and taken care of in-patients for close to fifty years, and I feel that despite the strides we have made in technology and medicine, we cannot let go of the fact that we are human and we have human needs that have to be addressed.

Hippocrates statement was "First, do no harm," and I think the future of medicine is hanging in that balance between technology and humanity. So *Speaking Up For Mom* draws attention to the fact that this is a person we are talking about and their experience can be much, much more positive if we all just wake up in the process. The doctors need to wake up, the nurses, the family and the individual. I think *Speaking Up For Mom* is helpful in alerting people to the possibilities.

Dr. Hanzelik On the Effectiveness of "Advance Directives"...

What is your impression of Advance Directives and do they really work?

I see Advance Directives as very valuable documents to help a person express their understanding that medical issues do happen and that they want to be prepared for them. In general, however, an Advance Directive doesn't work in a medical situation unless someone is there to push it, emphasize what's in it and make it clear to the appropriate people who carry out those decisions that this is what the patient wants. This becomes a major role on the part of the family member or their health care proxy - to make sure that the Advance Directives of the patient are carried out.

How effective is one Advance Directive, the "Living Will"?

The "Living Will" is an Advance Directive that describes what kind of medical care the person desires. So it's a legal document, but it's not the same as physician's medical orders. The only way to implement the details of the "Living Will" is through actual medical orders by a doctor.

Convey your experience with the POLST.

The POLST (Physician Orders for Life-Sustaining Treatment) is actual physician orders, and paramedics who come to a patient's house or hospitalists at the hospital are tuned in to respect the POLST. However, it differs from Advance Directives in that the POLST originates from the patient's physician rather than the patient. Basically, the doctor makes orders that say, "If this person has a cardiac arrest, I do not want you to do resuscitation on this patient." It's a medical order. I think the POLST works if it's available, and if it can be located when needed.

How about the DNR?

DNR (Do Not Resuscitate) is a medical order that also comes from the doctor and can be part of the POLST or exist by itself. For the hospital staff, the main question that is asked about a seriously-ill patient is, "Is this patient a DNR?" If the patient is a DNR, then that is labelled on the patient's chart and written everywhere in their records so that the medical staff knows not to call the cardiac team if the patient loses consciousness.

In the hospital, if a patient has a cardiac arrest, usually as soon as the nurses spot it, they immediately call the cardiac arrest team and that team (people who don't know the patient at all but are charged with doing resuscitations) will run into the room and start pounding on the patient's chest and putting a tube down the patient's throat to help them breathe - and do everything they can to resuscitate the patient. If the patient's chart is labeled DNR, however, and it's part of the physician's orders, then when the nurse sees this, she realizes this patient is a DNR and she won't call the resuscitation team. Typically in that situation, the nurse will first communicate what's on the chart to the doctor on call, who will then tell the nurse that the patient is a DNR.

It's important to understand one thing about the DNR. When a hospitalist looks at a critical situation, frequently they don't know the patient and don't want to make a mistake and let a person die who shouldn't be dying. So they always err on the side of doing everything they can to treat that person, unless someone speaks up and says this is not what that person wants. It needs to be very clear in order for the doctor to let the person go. Otherwise, the doctor feels that they are making a big mistake.

So the health care proxy needs to speak up when the patient is admitted, and say, "I'm this person's health care proxy. Here's a copy of the Advance Directive naming me. I'll be the contact person for you, and this person does not want excessive care." You can then have a conversation with the attending doctor about your loved one's code status. You can ask, "My loved one has requested to be "Do Not Resuscitate." Will you note that on the chart?" Then the doctor will initiate the DNR so the hospitalists will know whether the patient is a DNR or not, because if the patient is a DNR, it makes things simpler for the hospitalist. However, it's a difficult thing for patients and health care proxies to talk about and I've seen a lot of patients be resuscitated who should not have been. So it's an important dialog.

Are you saying there are times when the health care proxy knows what their loved one wants, and communicates that to the medical staff, and it is still not followed?

Yes, definitely. And that's when the health care proxy, having done their homework and relying on their own inner strength, is so crucial. The most serious thing that can happen is when someone is dying and the health care proxy says, "Do not resuscitate!" and the medical staff says, "We have to resuscitate!" and starts putting tubes down the patient's throat and pushing on their chest and putting the patient in the Intensive Care Unit. This happens because the medical staff is not convinced that the patient actually chose to be a "do not resuscitate" patient. We see this frequently, where the patient or proxy and the doctor are on a different page.

That's why the POLST is so helpful. It's an order from the doctor saying "do not resuscitate". But when there is someone just verbally saying it, without that doctor order backing it up, the hospital or the paramedics are in a position where they feel they have to protect themselves legally and they say, "Unless we are sure, we've got to resuscitate. Otherwise, someone will come back and say that we let a person die who shouldn't have died." So it can be very confusing in those last few critical minutes, and the clearer that the health care proxy is about their loved one's wishes, the better.

Therefore, a health care proxy can probably stop their loved one from having a medical procedure, but when it comes to life or death situations where resuscitation is happening, the health care proxy can yell stop and the staff will not stop?

Yes, because the medical staff may feel that they are legally liable. They might ask the health care proxy to show them the legal documents of POLST or DNR so they can review it. That's why it's better to have such physician orders in place and available before you get to those moments. However, if a critical situation is already in progress when the patient arrives at the hospital and the patient is arresting, only the POLST will slow down resuscitation at that point.

Dr. Hanzelik On Relieving the Patient's Suffering...

When, if ever, is it no longer up to the patient to decide their fate in the health care system, but is instead up to their health care proxy?

As we've talked about, the "Durable Power of Attorney for Health Care" is one of the Advance Directives that are usually drawn up by a lawyer and it designates the person's health care proxy. When to activate this document often depends on the patient's ability to make decisions. If the patient can think through a decision and ask appropriate questions and say, "Yes, I want to do this,"or "I don't want to do this," then it's the patient's decision.

But if the patient is unconscious, demented, unable to talk, or an emotional wreck or hysterical, then the doctor doesn't have someone they can work with to make meaningful decisions. Therefore, the responsibility goes to whomever the patient has legally designated for that role, or If they have not designated someone, then it goes to whomever seems to be the closest person in their family who is functioning in that role. Frequently, the proxy will bring in the patient's "Durable Power of Attorney for Health Care" document to the facility and show that their name is listed. If so, then that designation will be respected and the proxy's name will be noted on the patient's chart.

Another situation that can activate the health care proxy is when the patient has a large family and all the family members start asking the doctor questions at different times. The doctor may say, "I can only talk to one family member," and it becomes necessary to delegate someone who will be the contact person for that doctor and communicate to the rest of the family about what's happening. Again, if there is no health care proxy listed, then the doctor will talk to the most prominent person in the family - usually the spouse or an adult child.

As was mentioned in the story of *Speaking Up For Mom*, sometimes doctors talk to the proxy about the patient as if the patient isn't in the room. They do this when they feel the person really doesn't get what is going on, and it does happen that these conversations may not be very sensitive to the patient. Personally, I believe the patient has much more understanding of the conversation than the physician realizes.

Sometimes, is it unclear for the health care proxy about what decisions to make?

Yes, and that is something that should definitely be explained and clearly understood when a person chooses to be a health care proxy or thinks about having a proxy. The proxy is there to insure that what actually happens with the loved one is as closely aligned as possible to what the person would want. It's not about having someone with a completely different attitude take over and make the decisions. The patient and health care proxy need to understand this, and the proxy needs to know what the loved one would be happiest with and speak up when needed.

What should the health care proxy do when they can see clearly that the medical treatments proposed, although they may extend life, will result in further suffering?

These are not easy decisions. These are hard decisions. Definitely there are times when a doctor is presenting that surgery is a good idea and it will allow the patient to live. However, the health care proxy may be feeling, "I don't want to put my loved one through that suffering and pain and they are not going to live that long anyway." So that's when doing one's homework is so important. The proxy needs an understanding of what their loved one wants (and what other family members want is also helpful to take into consideration.)

Once the health care proxy is clear headed, he or she can stand up for what their loved one wants and the medical staff will listen to them. It can be very, very challenging at times, and the hospital is a rushed environment and everything is an emergency. So it's not easy to do this. But the more grounded the proxy is, the more knowledge they have, the more they understand their role, they can play a very important part in the decision-making.

Are there other resources available, in your opinion, to help someone be an effective health care proxy when they need to make a medical decision for a loved one?

The first resource is the relationship that you have with your or your loved one's primary care physician. In the story of *Speaking Up For Mom*, it sounds like this help really wasn't available during the mother's hospitalizations. However, when you do have that relationship, a primary care doctor will take the time to hear what your issues are, help you understand your options, and guide you so that you can make better choices and be more comfortable with the process. Otherwise, the process can seem to be constantly galloping ahead of you and you are always trying to play catch up.

If you don't have that support, the next best idea is to do your homework online before important medical decisions need to take place. I think there are more and more reliable resources that are coming online and developing, but you have to dig a little bit to find them. And it's important to find legitimate sources from people who have had experience and know what they are talking about.

Should the back-up proxy listed in the "Durable Health Power of Attorney" be kept in the loop about the loved one's care?

I think it is wise to have several back-up proxies listed in the "Durable Power of Attorney for Health Care" (most often the spouse and the adult children of the person). The first proxy can then make an effort to keep the other people in the loop. In an ideal situation, all the potential proxies love the person being protected. They communicate well. They all want to help.

In reality, there are often conflicts and lots of emotional baggage, including jealousy, resentment, anger among the parties, and issues emerge about the "Final Will and Testament." In addition, the burden of providing patient support often falls to one individual. So there is no "one size fits all" for these situations. Every person must find their way in responding to these challenging issues. My advice: things works out best when love, kindness, cooperation, caring and understanding are the foundation.

What is your impression of palliative care...Is it helpful? If so, how?

There's a recent distinction being made between "palliative care" and "hospice." It used to be that hospice *was* palliative care. Palliative care is basically, as I understand it, where the doctor is providing care - not to extend life or to cure the person or to help them get better - but accepting that they do have serious medical problems and the objective is for them to be as comfortable as possible in that process. So the doctor might more commonly use morphine or use medicines to relax the person, give medicines sublingually so that they don't need injections, and just focus on patient comfort rather than extending life. The objective is to try to be non-invasive so there's a lot things the doctor will not do - like dialysis, chemotherapy, big intravenous (PICC) lines and frequent blood tests. I don't think it's obvious yet what the nursing staff would do differently if the doctor just wrote down "palliative care"on the patient's chart. The doctor's orders need to be more specific. And it's not clear to me who would implement what changes in the patient's care. So I think palliative care is an indirect way of saying, "We are not going to resuscitate this patient."

Volandes' book *The Conversation* describes three levels of care that a patient needs to choose from. The first is "life sustaining care" where anything that will extend the person's life even a little bit is considered appropriate (i.e., intubation, intravenous drugs, artificial feeding.) The second level of care is "limited care" where the patient is willing to accept certain medical treatments to help their condition but there are certain very invasive treatments that they won't accept (i.e., intubation, feeding tubes, dialysis). These are things that the patient or doctor decides are more painful than beneficial and therefore, the physician accepts the fact that the patient may die if they limit care.

The third level is "comfort care," where the only focus is to keep the patient comfortable. The doctor is not really trying to extend life. The goal is just for the person to be comfortable and not be suffering. The book refers to this third option as palliative care - letting the person be in as good a shape as they can be and able to communicate as well as they can during the time that they have.

So I don't think the distinction between palliative care and hospice care is apparent yet. The hospice people understand the difference. But palliative care is just becoming a possibility in many places. Most hospitals feel as soon as a patient is on palliative or hospice care that the hospital has nothing more to offer the patient and the patient should leave.

What is the advantage of hospice for a critically ill or terminally ill patient, and what is the process whereby a patient is admitted to hospice by their primary care physician?

A determination of hospice for the patient makes everything clearer. A team of medical staff from outside the hospital or instead of the home medical care agency gets involved, and this team knows exactly what to do. They have their own doctors and use different kinds of medicines than acute care doctors use. They basically take over the patient care.

When a patient of mine is ready for hospice, I just write an order for a consultation with a hospice agency. Then the hospice agent comes and meets with the family, meets with the patient and comes back to me about whether the patient is appropriate for hospice. If the patient's health care proxy calls hospice directly, then hospice will call me and say that the patient has been evaluated and they feel that the patient is appropriate for hospice. But the patient's doctor definitely has a role to play, because it's usually the doctor to whom the patient's family talks to first, saying, "We think perhaps our loved one should be in hospice."

This gives the doctor an opportunity to say, "No, the patient doesn't need hospice." But if the family or proxy pushes a little bit, a hospice evaluation can be made available to people who want it and the hospice agency will make their own determination if the patient is eligible for hospice.

How can a hospital patient to be evaluated for hospice?

If your loved one is in the hospital, you can bring up hospice to whomever will listen to you. You can tell the hospital nurse, "I am interested in looking into hospice." Or you can talk to the admitting doctor at the facility. You can call the hospitalist at his or her office, instead of waiting for them to show up at the hospital. And, as I mentioned, if you are not getting a response from the hospitalist, you can call hospice yourself. You can ask the nurses at the hospital, "What is a good hospice?" There are a lot of different hospices available, and it's good to know which ones are recommended.

Then you can contact one or two of them and say, for instance, "My mother is in the hospital. I want to explore the possibility of hospice. How do I do this?" They will guide you through the process. At some point, the attending doctor needs to get involved because he or she needs to write the medical order for the patient to be on hospice. You are initiating the evaluation but the doctor needs to approve it. And, yes, Medicare will cover it. Hospice won't accept the patient unless Medicare covers it.

Suppose the doctor is resistant to a patient being accepted into hospice?

Hospices are private agencies, somewhat like home health care agencies, and sometimes they are even part of a home health care agency. So you can look up local hospices in the phone directory or online and you'll find a list. Then you can just call and say, "My loved one is experiencing this, this and this, and I'm concerned that he/she needs to be in hospice," and they will guide you through the process.

It's possible the hospice might say, "Well, have you spoken to the patient's doctor yet?" And if you say no, that the doctor didn't seem to want to talk about it, they might say. "Well, talk to the doctor first and then get back to us." But my impression is that hospice is willing to do the evaluation. I've seen it many times. Patients of mine have ended up in hospice who I didn't even know were applying to hospice at the time. So I think the process is flexible. And people who qualify for hospice need to be there. The only thing the doctor has to declare in order for them to be admitted to hospice and for the government to pay for it is that the patient's life expectancy is six months or less. However, I do have patients in hospice who have been alive for a long period of time and are doing fine.

Please relate the story about your mother passing away. It's a sweet example of speaking up for your loved one.

My mother smoked cigarettes her whole life and she never wanted any part of medical care. She didn't like the idea of doctors and she avoided seeing them completely. So when she finally did go to the hospital, her condition was extremely advanced. She had a huge mass in her spleen which turned out to be a lymphoma.

I went to see her in the hospital and she was terrified. She never liked hospitals because she said the doctors were coming at her from every direction with needles. (She hated the little needles they used for blood tests and for tests under the skin.) And one thing she said to me was, "How do I die?" because she knew she was dying. I just told her, "It's a natural thing. It will happen when it happens. You don't have to do anything." In fact, I don't think she was too concerned about it.

Yet, as I've mentioned, I saw how she perceived that people were coming at her with needles from all directions. So the one great thing I did say to her was, "It's your choice. It's completely your choice. If you want this treatment or not, or if you want to stay in the hospital or not, it's your choice." And it was like a light bulb went off in her head and she immediately decided that she wanted to go home.

The surgeon had already opened her up and decided it was too late to do anything. So, the hospital really had nothing to offer except to make her pretty miserable while she waited for her doctors to reach the same conclusion. So she was very relieved to go home. And we had hospice work with her and in a lot of ways it worked out very beautifully. My sister was there and it was a much better situation for my mother.

One day, after she left the hospital, my wife and I took her for a ride in our car and while we were riding, we told her we would grant her three wishes. Her first wish was that she wanted someone with her at all times to take care of her - which was a good wish and we implemented that fairly quickly. The second wish was that she wanted a Cadillac, and I wish we had implemented that one a little quicker than we did. Her third wish was that she wanted a divorce from my father. They were always fighting with each other and he could be obnoxious at times. It had become a frustrating situation for her, besides the fact that my father was getting a little demented. So we implemented more separation between them and more privacy. They were in the same house but they had their own rooms and my father wasn't around as much as before, so her needs were able to be more easily addressed.

Throughout her whole life, my mother had been dealing with depression. When she was eight years old, her older sister had died and that had a life-long effect on my mother. So it was surprising that my mother was so at peace with dying. In fact, the hospice staff said her death was one of the most peaceful they had ever witnessed.

"Nine

Important

"Lessons"

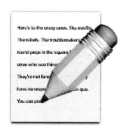

This section is a reference guide
for the topics covered
in "Mom's Story" and "The Doctor Is In."

"I feel the most important factor in the outcome of care is the clarity and strength of the caregivers and the people making the medical decisions to do what's best for the patient. But the medical environment is quite intimidating and the decision makers need support and even training to handle their responsibilities effectively."

— Dr. Hanzelik

Lesson 1: Find Out What You Don't Know

We have nine months to prepare for birth. With death, it varies. Most of us don't want to think about it or talk about it, especially with our loved ones. I get it. It's painful. But, then, so is the alternative of operating in a "crisis orientation."

Mom and I never had the all-important conversation about her end-of-life care. The few times I broached the subject, she wouldn't hear of it. Perhaps, this was partly due to her prior experience with doctors, but my own lack of understanding about how to start the conversation didn't help.

Regardless of the reason, I found myself coming to her aid near the end of her life with no idea of what she wanted - although indirectly she tried to tell me. And once she was admitted to the hospital, I unconsciously activated my authority as her health care proxy, with no hesitation from her doctors, and took away her power to choose. At the time, it just seemed easier and more expedient that way. Looking back, I think it was a huge mistake.

It's clear to me now why it's so important to talk with your loved one about their health care wishes *before* a health crisis occurs. I should have sought out the advice I needed to overcome my fear of rejection and have this conversation with Mom. If you find yourself in a similar circumstance, I encourage you to do what I did not. . .

A Guided Conversation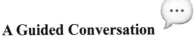

Sometimes it's difficult for a family member to bring up the subject of end-of-life care. This is when it may be helpful to bring in a friend, a clergy, a doctor or other person whom the loved one trusts, in order to facilitate the conversation.

 One important thing to point out is that the conversation itself should be more like an interview than a discussion. Its purpose is not to try to persuade your loved one to think your way or to do what you want them to do. Remember, this is their life and you are there only as a support. Avoid judging or steering their answers.

Below are just a few of many important questions that can help guide this interaction. Many such lists are available. This excerpt is from "Conversations That Light the Way" by The Ohio End of Life Collaborative [1]:

❑ How important is it for you to be able to care for yourself? (very important, somewhat important, not important)

❑ What kind of living environment would you be willing to accept? (assisted living, retirement village, private apartment, nursing facility, extended care facility)

❑ What does very advanced age mean to you?

❑ Do you fear any particular treatments or procedures?

❑ If you have a memory of a loved one's death, what did you learn from that experience?

❑ What beliefs do you hold that influence your thoughts about life and about dying?

❑ Would you want treatments that might prolong your life (ex., tube feedings) if you were: comatose and not likely to regain consciousness; terminally ill or near death?

❑ What important needs would you want to be addressed if you were dying?

❑ What are your fears or concerns about the end of life?

Lesson 2: Make the Most of a Doctor Visit

In Chapter Two of the story, I mentioned that I noticed a slightly different approach to Mom's care from doctors in Florida compared to those in Ohio. The situation in Florida was far from ideal, but physicians there appeared to take her age and medical issues into consideration when prescribing (or not prescribing) certain long-range treatments and medications. I assume this was due more to their frequent interaction with Mom's age group rather than to any specialized training that they had.

Yet, toward the end of Mom's life, I began to wish all of her doctors understood more about how to treat a woman in her eighties who had a chronic, ultimately terminal condition (congestive heart failure) and who had no desire to live as an invalid. I now know that there were things I could have done to improve the situation. Let's discuss some of these.

An Effective Doctor Visit

As your loved one's caregiver or health care proxy, it's important to make the most of their doctor visits. The average time a doctor spends with a patient is only seven minutes, so here are some things you can do to make the most of that precious time:

❏ Request a "well" visit for your loved one before health issues arise. This will give the doctor a "baseline" of what's normal for the patient to compare against in case a health issue arises. For instance, evidence is mounting that the elderly are more likely to have "normal" blood pressures above what's considered normal for younger adults. The American Geriatrics Society says attempting to lower the blood pressure of elderly patients to the standard "normal" using medication has not shown to reduce their risk of dying.[2]

❏ Make a list of all the medical symptoms you or your loved
   one are concerned about. Then do some investigating online
   at reputable websites to get a list of possible diagnoses,
   just as a starting point for conversation with the physician.
   Some recommended websites include **WebMD.com** and
   ClevelandClinic.com.

❏ Call ahead to request a phone appointment with the doctor or
   nurse if you have any concerns about your loved one's health
   that you don't feel comfortable discussing in their presence; or
   leave a message asking the doctor to bring up those concerns
   with your loved one at their next appointment.

❏ Trust your judgment and insist on further examination if you
   feel something is wrong that is not being detected or addressed.
   Remember that you or anyone who spends significant time with
   your loved one knows more about their symptoms, health issues
   or changes in behavior than a doctor who spends minutes with
   the patient every few months.

❏ Take notes! This will reduce your loved one's anxiety about
   having to remember what is said, and it will also give you some
   discussion points to review with them after the appointment.

Shared Decision Making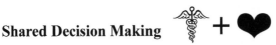

A new concept in the doctor-patient relationship is called "Shared
Decision Making" or SDM. Much of the time that doctors previously
spent getting to know their patients has evaporated due to increased case
loads, physician group pressures and less reimbursement from insurers.
Because of this, there can be a noticeable decline in the quality of care. To
bridge this gap, **Shared Decision Making** intends to:

✚ strengthen communication between the health care provider and the
   patient

✚ provide better decision making about treatment options

✚ take into account the health priorities and quality-of-life goals of the patient

Everyone from *The New England Journal of Medicine* to the Mayo Clinic to the U.S. government is touting the benefits of SDM. In fact, the Mayo Clinic has even created the "Mayo Clinic Shared Decision Making National Resource Center" to help physicians understand the process, as one of the main obstacles to widespread use of SDM is that doctors are traditionally not trained to communicate in this way.

Q. What specific benefits does the patient receive with Shared Decision Making?

A. The "Shared Decision Making Fact Sheet," from healthit.gov, explains that with SDM, a patient will:

✔ learn about their health and understand their health conditions

✔ recognize that a decision needs to be made and be informed about the options

✔ understand the pros and cons of different options

✔ have the information and tools needed to evaluate their options

✔ be better prepared to talk with their health care provider

✔ collaborate with their health care team to make a decision right for them

✔ be more likely to follow through on their decision

Along with the above, SDM also:

✚ *reaffirms* a patient's right to access their own medical records (see "Who's Heard of HIPPA?", page 112);

✚ *encourages* the patient to ask questions;

✚ *stresses* full disclosure of information to the patient in order to weigh treatment options;

✚   *lays out statistics* about survival rates, cure rates, etc. of treatment;

✚   *utilizes informed consent* when agreeing to an invasive treatment plan.
     (See "Is There Something Called Patient Rights?", Lesson 3.)

A perspective in the *New England Journal of Medicine* expresses the
potential of SDM this way [3]:

> *"...shared decision making will require clinicians to work
> against their natural impulses to tell the patient what to do
> when they're certain of what's best, and to leave the patient to
> decide when they're not. 'I'm not sure what the right answer is,
> so why don't you decide' can be replaced with, 'This is a really
> hard decision because we aren't sure what will happen if you
> choose option x; let me show you how I think about this, and
> you can tell me whether it fits with what's important to you.'
> And, equally important, 'I'm recommending option x because it
> provides better outcomes than option y' can become, 'Let me tell
> you about the pros and cons of options x and y so that you can
> decide which one matches your priorities.'"*

You can download the "Shared Decision Making Factsheet" at
healthit.gov and share it with your loved one's physician to find
out their position on shared decision making. If you or your loved
one feels that their physician will not participate in share decision
making; or hasn't the expertise to work well with the elderly; or
you are uncomfortable with their "bedside manner;" there are
some other possibilities below.

What is Geriatrics?

Geriatrics is a specialized field of medicine that deals with the health
problems of the elderly. It offers board certified internists and family
physicians the option of an additional one to two years of training to
become geriatricians.

Q. When is seeking out a geriatrician most beneficial?

A. The American Geriatrics Society says primary care provided by a geriatrician rather than a family care physician may be especially beneficial when:

- the patient's medical condition is in a frail or weakened state;

- the patient is older than seventy-five and has several medical issues including mental impairment;

- or the caregiver(s) is feeling overwhelmed by their caregiver situation with the elderly person.

Another helpful specialty for the aged is a subset of psychiatry called *geriatric psychiatry* or *psychogeriatrics*. It deals with the mental issues of patients over age sixty-five, including delirium and dementia.

Not to be confused with geriatrics, *gerontology* is a health profession that specializes in care of the elderly. However, a gerontologist is usually *not* a licensed physician and may not even work directly with patients. They study how to increase the quality of life of the elderly through research, public policy or other ways.

 A list of geriatricians can be found at websites like **healthinaging.org** which links to the American Geriatrics Society database with search capability. Simply type in your state to find a geriatrician near you.

 Lessons 4 and 8 describe in greater detail why this expertise may be useful when deciding about drug therapies and medical procedures for an elderly patient.

Examining "Physician Groups"

Doctors typically see 40-50 patients a day and most are part of a "physicians' group" where several doctors band together to cut operating (billing) and liability (insurance) costs. These groups are more the norm than ever, with only 40% of U.S. primary care physicians currently owning and operating their own practice.[4]

One challenge of using a physicians' group is getting an appointment when it's needed on short notice. Most doctors book appointments months in advance. Consequently if there's an emergency or urgent situation, the patient is directed to the emergency room or an urgent care clinic. And if the patient does manage to get an appointment with their doctor, they often end up seeing a physician's assistant, not the doctor. Dr. Hanzelik says these doctors are also required to recommend a specialist within their group if one is needed - even if that specialist may not be the best choice for the patient. Parents of the Baby Boomer generation or even Baby Boomers themselves grew up under the care of family doctors who were well acquainted with their patients' health histories and even recalled such personal details as which colleges their children attended. Thus, many of these patients are dissatisfied with the service of physician groups and are looking for alternatives in their health care. For this reason, personalized or "concierge" medical groups are coming into view.

"Personalized" Physician Services

Personalized or concierge medical groups are groups of physicians who have decided that they want to make preventative health care their first priority, promote wellness, focus on customer and patient care, and personalize medical care for their patients. These groups want to:

+ be available to their patients 24/7, without enlisting a call-in service or referring to another doctor on the weekends

+ allow their patients to make same day appointments

+ encourage patients to engage in their own health care

+ advocate for the patient in the hospital by conferring with the hospital physicians ("hospitalists")

+ do home visits, if needed!

So, how are these personalized physician groups able to do what a typical physician group cannot? Physician group doctors have an average case load of 2000-2500 patients, plus they often take on the care of one or more rehabilitation or nursing care facilities to supplement their income. Personalized physician groups, on the other hand, typically care for a quarter of that number, which gives them more time to get to know each patient. But to enlist their services, these doctors must charge a monthly fee that patients pay above and beyond their health insurance costs.[5]

Integrative Medicine, A New Alternative

Often, traditional Western medicine in the U.S. focuses on acute care (quick fixes) and symptom relief, but rarely undertakes the more time-consuming process of focusing on the healing potential of the "whole person," i.e., exploring possible disease promoting factors such as the patient's mental state, environmental conditions, family health history, nutritional status, lifestyle habits or sudden life events which can have a profound effect on one's health. However, healing modalities outside the parameters of conventional medicine do exist and some do try to address these factors. Such forms of treatment may include:

+ acupuncture

+ nutritional counseling

+ osteopathic manipulation

+ chiropractic

+ stress management

+ homeopathy

+ herbal medicine

Also known as complimentary and alternative medicine (CAM), integrative medicine is now the preferred term for this approach as defined by The Academy of Integrative Health & Medicine. It refers to "a broad range of healing philosophies and approaches that are outside of conventional approaches but can be used as stand-alone alternatives or adjunctive approaches to conventional care."

The trend is that more and more conventionally trained physicians and hospitals are offering some kind of integrative medicine services. If your loved one, like my mom, has a basic mistrust of conventional medicine, this might be a possible alternative. Just be aware that working with a person's innate healing properties takes time and, unlike traditional Western medicine, may require patience to find the right combination of healing practices that work for the patient.

It is common practice for physician practices and medical screening and laboratory facilities that typically accept medical insurance to offer a discount, at times substantial, to patients who do not have insurance or their insurance policy denies the claim and the patient must pay for the service out of pocket. If you are ever in that circumstance, contact the service provider before paying their bill. A payment schedule can also often be arranged.

 On the academy's website **aihm.org**, you can find a list of integrative medicine practitioners throughout the U.S. Not all those listed are M.D.s, some are not accepting new patients, and some do not accept major health insurance plans. However, this list can be a starting point.

Who's Heard of HIPAA?

Have you ever watched a doctor or nurse type notes into your loved one's medical file and wished you could see what they were writing? Or have you felt like there was a mysterious medical diary following your loved one throughout their healthcare journey that you were not privy too? I know I did. I had no idea I could access these documents about Mom and learn more about what she was being tested for, and what her true prognosis was.

In 1996, a law was passed by the U.S. Congress called the "Health Insurance Portability and Accountability Act" (HIPAA) that effectively addressed this issue. It established a "bill of rights" regarding patient medical records and it contains two important sections - the Right to Access and the Privacy Rule. It's important to get familiar with both.

HIPAA'S Right to Access

The purpose of HIPAA's Right to Access is to guarantee that a person has access to their Protected Health Information (PHI) generated by any health insurance plan or health care provider; and that this information be made available to the patient as long as the business entity stores these records.

PHI includes all the information in any form that is used for diagnosis, treatment or payment regarding a person's medical records, such as:

- lab results

- clinical case notes

- medical program files

- billing and payment records

In most cases, request for this information need not be in writing, and access must be made available within 30 days, if not sooner. Also, you do not need to provide a reason for your request, and outstanding medical bills cannot be used as a reason for denial. If for some reason your request is denied (which is rare) the denial can be sent to an oversight body for review.

Providing PHI information allows for greater understanding by the patient regarding their treatment plans and progress - and its cost. It is considered integral to a person's health care and should be provided for free. If a paper version of the report is requested, small fees are allowed to cover printing, mailing and administrative costs.

Medicare and Medicaid have a program called the Electronic Health Records (EHR) Incentive Program which gives incentive payments to health care providers and hospitals using the EHR technology. This encourages them to allow patients to view online, download and transmit their own health information. A summary of the PHI, rather than the information itself, can be made available for a fee.

Q. Is anything omitted from a patient's PHI report?

A. Yes. The report does not include information which may be used in ways other than to treat the individual, such as:

- an institution's quality assessments

- business planning or management activities in the business entity

- psychotherapy notes taken in therapy sessions

- information compiled for use in a legal proceeding.

However, any individual information used to generate those reports is available to the patient.

 The website **medicare.gov/physiciancompare** lists about 860,000 U.S. physicians along with information such as:
- their hospital affiliation
- whether they accept Medicare
- whether they are part of a group practice
- do they participate in programs such as the EHR

HIPPA's Privacy Rule

Q. Who, besides the patient, has access to their medical records?

A. This is where the HIPAA Privacy Rule comes in. The idea behind it is that others won't have access to the PHI without the patient's permission, *with these exceptions:*

- when a patient engages a health care provider, medical facility or health insurance plan, the patient usually signs something giving that entity permission to access their entire PHI.

- the patient's health care proxy also automatically has access.

- the patient can also designate a family member or anyone else to have access to their PHI, but this must be done in writing.

 For more detailed information and Q&A about HIPAA, see the U.S. Dept. of Health and Human Services website at **hhs.gov/hipaa/for-professionals/privacy/guidance/access**.

Lesson 3: Be Their Voice

When Mom became a widow, she had her "Last Will and Testament" revised by her Florida lawyer, and she asked me sign a legal document called a "Durable Power of Attorney for Health Care". Once she moved to Ohio and my caregiving became more frequent, I began carrying a copy of this document with me in case I ever needed it. However, I never read it closely or familiarized myself with its contents. All I knew was that it had something to do with representing her in a medical emergency, in case she couldn't represent herself.

When you sign that document, your loved one breathes a sigh of relief. Now they know someone with their best interests at heart will be in control of what happens to them medically, should they ever need it, and perhaps save them from unwanted tests and procedures that could turn them into a human pin cushion.

But in reality, most of us don't know what our authority or role is when it comes to acting as someone's health care proxy. At least, I know I didn't. And I soon learned that the medical establishment is not required nor likely to explain it to you. So let's learn what it means to sign that "Durable Power of Attorney for Health Care" to designate your own or to become someone else's health care proxy.

What Are Advance Directives?

As important as it is to have a guided conversation with your loved one regarding their medical care preferences, it is equally important to legally cover those situations where your loved one cannot personally communicate those wishes in a medical setting, either due to their medical condition or their mental state. This is where "Advance Directives" comes in.

Advance Directives is typically a set of three legal documents that gives direction to those charged with the patient's well being, about how to proceed - or the limits on how to proceed - with medical care based on the patient's wishes.

☛ *The patient may change these directives at any time as long as he or she is mentally competent, however, the changes must be done in writing.*

Q. What are the three documents of the Advance Directives?

A. The first is called the "Durable Power of Attorney for Health Care." It designates someone as the person's health care agent, health care proxy, health care surrogate, health care representative or health care attorney-in-fact. According to the National Institutes of Health, a health care agent or proxy is "someone you choose to make health care decisions for you when you cannot." There are three important things to note about appointing a health care proxy:

✔ The patient is the one who decides who will speak on their behalf and be their legal authority;

✔ The proxy's authority covers only issues related to the patient's health care, nothing else (i.e., financial decisions);

✔ The proxy's responsibility occurs only when the patient is physically or mentally incapable of making their own healthcare decisions. (And this is determined by evaluation from at least one physician.)

Q. Is this first Advance Directive always needed?

A. The short answer is "no." It is not needed when:

- a parent is automatically a health care proxy for their own child

- a spouse is automatically considered the health proxy for their marriage partner

However, circumstances where they will be needed include:

- you want your adult child to be your backup health care proxy

- or a single person wants their adult child to be their proxy;

- or a child over the age of eighteen wants their parents to be their health care proxy,

Check with legal counsel in your state to be sure.

 Find more information online about being a health care proxy at
talk-early-talk-often.com/medical-power-of-attorney.html

Q. What are the responsibilities of a health care proxy?

**A. Being a health care proxy for a child is somewhat different that
being one for an adult.** For a child, we most likely make decisions
based on what we feel are in their best interests. *For an adult, our role
is to carry out the patient's wishes, whether we agree with those wishes
or not.* The "Durable Power of Attorney for Health Care" document
empowers the health care proxy to make a wide-range of health care
decisions for their loved one, including (from lawhelp.org):

✔ whether to admit or discharge the patient from a hospital or nursing
home;

✔ which treatments or medicines you do or do not want them to receive;

✔ who has access to their medical records.

Sounds like pretty far-reaching powers, doesn't it? It is. Regardless
of any other input or advice from family members or physicians or legal
counsel, the health care proxy named in this document has the final say on
your loved one's care when they cannot speak for themselves. That is…
with perhaps one *important* exception.

Q. Is the "Living Will" the second Advance Directive?

**A. Yes. In the Living Will, the patient gives direction *in writing*
regarding his/her medical care in case they are unable to
communicate it at the time it's needed.** This document allows the
patient to specify their preferences regarding critical treatment options
such as:

- cardiopulmonary resuscitation (CPR)

- artificially supplied nutrition or hydration

- mechanical ventilation

- dialysis

- antibiotics in a terminal illness

- palliative care (see "Lesson 8: Know When Enough Is Enough")

The Living Will must be witnessed and signed by someone other than the patient's blood relative, health care provider or health care proxy.

> *Instructions in the Living Will are meant to override the Durable Power of Attorney for Health Care in most cases, even if the patient is unconscious, mentally incompetent or unable to communicate. Make sure a copy of both your loved one's Living Will and Durable Power of Attorney for Health Care are on file with their physician and/or the medical facility where they are admitted.*

Again, as their health care proxy, read and be familiar with those directives yourself! You are the protector of your loved one's medical wishes, so if others insist that everything possible be done to save the person and that is not their wish, know who you can call on for support, i.e., the primary care physician, other relative, etc.

Q. What is the third document of the Advance Directives?

A. It can vary, depending on the state of jurisdiction. For example, it may be an Organ Donor form or a Guardianship Nomination form, in case that is ever needed.

> *A Living Will is not the same thing as a "Final Will and Testament" which is used to manage a person's estate after their death.*

Q. Where can I find "Advance Directives" forms?

A. Legal forms for Advance Directives can be obtained for free from many different sources:

- a local hospital

- online at **americanbar.org** or other legal form websites

- routinely included in attorney services for a "Last Will and Testament."

> The website **caringinfo.org** has a button on its homepage, "Download Your State Specific Advance Directive." It links to a downloadable version of Advance Directive forms for every U.S. state.

Q. Are there "doctor generated" advance directives?

A. Yes. There are two. The first is "Do Not Resuscitate" or DNR. This is a physician or medical facility provided order that allows individuals to make decisions about their own emergency medical treatment.

DNR came into being as part of the Patient Self-Determination Act of 1991. According to **medlineplus.gov**, a website of the National Institutes of Health,

> "A do-not-resuscitate order, or DNR order, is a medical order written by a doctor. It instructs health care providers not to do cardiopulmonary resuscitation (CPR) if a patient's breathing stops or if a patient's heart stops beating...It does not have instructions for other treatments such as pain medicines, other medicines or nutrition."

Sounds pretty intense, doesn't it? It is...There's no going back if this order is signed by the doctor and followed, unless the health care proxy is physically there in time to reverse it. So why have the doctor sign it? Many patients don't want to have their lives extended artificially or to be kept alive in a vegetative state, or to have extreme measures taken to save themselves. It's especially relevant to the elderly who may wish to die a natural death and for whom the survival rate from cardiac pulmonary resuscitation (CPR) in a hospital setting is often statistically low.[6]

Q. If a DNR is *not* signed by the doctor, what happens when medical personnel or trained first responders attempt to resuscitate someone?

A. The Ohio Department of Health "Do Not Resuscitate (DNR): Frequently Asked Questions[7]," states resuscitative treatment typically includes:

- chest compressions

- electric heart shock

- an artificial breathing tube down the throat (intubation)

- special drugs delivered via an arm 'IV port'

So, if your loved one wants to avoid this, *the DNR must be SIGNED by the patient's doctor - either the hospitalist at the medical facility or the family physician if the patient is living at home. Without it, the DNR is void and will not be carried out,* unless you, as the health care proxy, are present to say otherwise and even then, a doctor's order will be required. As you know from Mom's story, I was remiss in getting her DNR signed at both facilities where she was admitted for rehabilitation. And in both cases, we needed it. My advice: hound the doctor until it is signed!

Q. What is the patient's or health care proxy's role in getting the DNR signed by their physician?

A. The DNR must first be signed by the patient or their health care proxy. If you've ever been with someone who is admitted to a hospital or a rehabilitation facility, you know the paperwork that ensues. It's almost like closing on a house sale! Among the stack of papers to sign (or not) is the DNR. It may look like just one more legal form, but actually it could be the most important paper you or your loved one signs. So it needs careful consideration before either of you pick up that pen.

Obviously, the DNR is extremely important to discuss with your loved one, if you are able to. If that's not possible, look carefully at their other life choices, e,g., the way they handled their own parents' or spouse's ending years or their general view of life and quality of life. All of these things will help draw a picture of what to do. I can tell you from having been in the position of signing the DNR for Mom that it is far from easy to uphold, even if all the paperwork is in place. But once the health care proxy knows what their loved one wants, either directly or through a gut feeling, it's up to the proxy to see that it is carried out.

Finally, if the decision is for the patient or proxy to sign it, ask when the doctor will see it and also sign it.

 Request a copy of the physician-signed DNR form to verify that it has been done, and keep a copy with you in case of emergency. For instance, it may be needed if the EMTs are called to a private home or a nursing home. In most states, if the signed DNR is not readily available, the EMTs will not wait for it.

 More information about the DNR is available as "DNR FAQ" in the "Helpful Resources" section of this book.

Q. What is the second "doctor generated" Advance Directive?

A. It is called the POLST or MOLST (Physician Orders for Life-Sustaining Treatment, Provider Orders for Life-Sustaining Treatment, or Medical Orders for Life-Sustaining Treatment). It is specifically designed as a "prescription" by the doctor for the treatment of seriously ill patients in an emergency situation. It is based on the patient's Advance Directives, treatment preferences and consultations with their doctor.

In 1991, this new accompaniment to the Advance Directives appeared on the medical scene and it is now being supported in some states throughout the U.S. The POLST organization, National POLST Paradigm, describes the purpose of the form as *"to ensure that, in case of an emergency, you receive the treatment you prefer."* It is filled out by the attending doctor and is prominently displayed near the patient's bed in a medical facility or if at home, where emergency teams can easily find it (on the refrigerator is a good place.)

Q. How is POLST or MOLST different from a DNR?

A. The POLST is a doctor's order, including the DNR and is posted at the patient's bedside. It is readily available at an instant and is not to be questioned. It also goes into greater detail about specific medications and treatment options.

Q. Why does a person need a POLST if they have a Living Will?

A. Often the Living Will is not filed with the facility in question or is not available at the time of need, so it often goes unheeded. Also, a POLST is a doctor's order indicating what Advance Directives have been created and who serves as the health care proxy. It can also go into more detail than the Living Will, detailing:

✔ requests not to transfer to an emergency room or not to be admitted to a hospital;

✔ what treatments not to use;

✔ when certain treatments can be used;

✔ how long such treatments can be used;

✔ and when the treatments should be stopped.

In general, it's easier for advance directives and DNRs to be complied with during the day, when there are more supervisors and staff available to back up those decisions and work with the family. However, during an emergency or a sudden change in the patient's condition that happens at, say, three a.m., when the attending doctor is not available and the situation requires an immediate response, the POLST OR MOLST is very useful as a concrete back up to the health care proxy caught off guard by the emergency who may be in shock and needing support for what their loved one wants in their health care.

 Like any Advance Directive, the content of the POLST can be cancelled or updated at the patient's or their health care proxy's request as the patient's medical condition changes or improves.

Q. Do Advance Directives really work?

A. The answer depends on who you ask. An article in *ACEP NOW,* a publication of the American College of Emergency Physicians, stated these "limitations," among others, of why Advance Directives don't always work in a hospital setting [8]:

- Their use (POLST for example) has been mandated but not funded

- There is no standardization or clarification of terms

- There is variable understanding among providers

- The forms are often not available at the time of need

- Informed discussion needs to take place in the primary care physician's office

According to this article, some institutions have adopted the "resuscitation pause" which "combines the ABC's (Airways, Breathing, Circulation) of resuscitation and a hospital process called the "Time out, or surgical pause." This means, once the doctor has stabilized the patient, there is a pause that allows the doctor and the patient or health care proxy to discuss the next steps based on the patient's POLST or individualized plan of care, the patient's health goals and their Advance Directives.

 One thing to consider about POLST and its use or lack thereof is in medical facilities run by certain religious organizations. Sometimes their religious teachings regarding end of life may reinforce the staff's reluctance to discontinue artificial life support, even if it is specified in a POLST. For this reason, the use of POLST may not be financially or institutionally supported at some of these facilities.

Q. Are there other reasons Advance Directives might not ensure that the patient's wishes will be carried out?

A. Yes. If the document is not readily available at the time of an emergency, even confirming that the physician has signed off on a POLST or DNR does not guarantee that it will be complied with. Also, sometimes in the midst of life or death situations, the health care proxy or family members are in shock and say, "Do whatever the doctor thinks!" This needs to change if we want to have more respectful outcomes for our loved ones.

When I was in this situation with Mom, I psychologically handed over my responsibility as her health care proxy and allowed her doctors to call the shots, which they were very willing to do. I understand now that I facilitated this by not understanding my power and rights as her health care proxy. Truthfully, the medical staff works for us and should listen to us, but this requires a paradigm shift on our part to have the appropriate paperwork available and to be ready to utilize it. Therefore, the role and dedication of the health care proxy to be prepared and speak up when needed is crucial for the critically or terminally ill patient.

 The intent of POLST is to let natural death occur if death is eminent. This is not the same as "Death With Dignity" legislation in which "physician aid-in-dying" or "physician assisted suicide" is allowed by prescribing medicines to hasten death. Even with a POLST, however, a signed "Do Not Resuscitate" order is needed in the event of cardiac arrest to specify that CPR not to be initiated.

 You can go to **polst.org/programs-in-your-state/** to see if your state has a POLST program. If not, you can advocate for one by contacting your elected officials or state medical association.

 A sample POLST [9] *is located in the "Helpful Resources" section of this book.*

Does Elder Law Help?

When Mom lived in Florida, she filed her Advance Directives with her local attorney. But when she moved to Ohio, I assumed these documents needed to be updated, so I took her to an Ohio Wills and Probate lawyer. Though everything was routine and we really weren't changing anything, she reacted with suspicion about the whole process, and the attorney visits and the signing of new documents proved to be traumatic for her. Much later, I learned that her Florida documents would have been sufficient and legally binding in Ohio. Unfortunately, my attorney never mentioned this to me and I didn't know to ask.

Q. How may Elder Law help?

A. It is a specialty within the legal field that deals with a broad range of concerns that affect the elderly including:

- Medicare/Medicaid payments

- Social security and long-term health insurance claims

- guardianships

- estate planning and transfer of assets

- retirement benefits

- management of trusts and long-term care placements

- Last Will and Testaments and Advance Directives

Most Elder Law attorneys specialize in only a few of these areas, so it's important to identify what expertise you or your loved one requires and then find attorneys in your area who have that expertise. Besides being more familiar with the local and state laws regarding the issues mentioned above, elder law attorneys are often more attuned to working with the elderly or those with dementia, and are familiar with the challenges of eldercare planning. They are also often connected to other resources that can be helpful for their clients or their caregivers.

The most important thing in selecting an elder law attorney is that they be someone you and your loved one trust and feel comfortable with, and who is open to answering your questions.

According to the Caregiver Action Network at **caregiveraction.org**, here are some questions to ask when determining whether to hire an elder law attorney:

❑ How much do you charge? Is there a retainer? Do you provide an initial free consultation?

❑ What is your level of experience dealing with situations like mine?

❑ What information should I prepare or bring to our first meeting?

❑ How long will it take to handle our situation?

❑ Will you be handling this matter yourself or will you be passing all or some on to another attorney?

❑ What documents do you recommend that I have in place to deal with my loved one's health care issues?

❑ Are there any specific issues I should be aware of because I live in/my loved one lives in _____(name of your state) ?

❑ Do I need my loved one(s) present when we talk?

❑ My loved one is moving to another state. Are their existing documents still valid or do we need to change them?

It is recommended to get any financial arrangement with an elder law attorney put into writing, so there are no surprises. In general, elder care lawyers can be expensive.

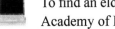 To find an elder law attorney near you, you can visit The National Academy of Elder Law Attorneys at **naela.org**.

Is There Something Called Patient Rights?

Our discussion of Advance Directives or how to represent or be represented by a health care proxy, would not be complete without touching on something called **"patient rights"**. It seems logical that patient rights would be enumerated somewhere, doesn't it? Actually, there's not much documentation on the subject. A few rights are guaranteed by the federal government (see HIPAA in Lesson 2.) States also determine their own patient rights, as do hospitals and medical facilities. These are often posted as a "Patient Bill of Rights" on obscure bulletin boards and are buried in the documents that a patient signs when retaining their medical services. But, as mentioned earlier, medical personnel are not required nor are likely to tell you what your rights are, so you must speak up if you want your rights or those of your loved one to be acknowledged.

Q. How important is "Informed Consent"?

A. Informed consent is at the core of patient rights and Shared Decision Making, especially when the physician is recommending a new plan of invasive treatment (see "Lesson 4: First, Do No Harm".) The American Cancer Society describes informed consent in this way:

✔ You are told (or get information in some way) about the possible risks and benefits of the treatment.

✔ You are told about the risks and benefits of other options, including not getting treatment.

✔ You have the chance to ask questions and get them answered to your satisfaction.

✔ You have had time (if needed) to discuss the plan with family or advisors.

✔ You are able to use the information to make a decision that you think is in your own best interest.

☛ *Make sure you get all your questions answered to your satisfaction before agreeing to any treatment. Do not abdicate this right, no matter how "inconvenient" it may seem for the medical staff.*

Lesson 4: First, Do No Harm

The phrase "First, do no harm," is often quoted when referring to the "Hippocratic Oath" which doctors take when they become physicians. Yet, it can also apply to the health care proxy.

Anyone who has been a caregiver for an elderly person knows the myriad of prescription medications and routine procedures that often accompany their loved one. For instance, by the time Mom arrived in Ohio and we enlisted her new doctors, she had an array of new pills to take, some of which required fasting or to be taken at specific times of the day. In addition, there were weekly blood tests for one of her medications and numerous follow-up doctor appointments scheduled at three month intervals.

Mom initially balked at the idea of taking prescription meds. When she finally gave in, she would intently scan the labels of her pill bottles as if they were poison. Overwhelmed with managing her care, I thought questioning every order from every doctor would be one more layer of complication. So to expedite things, I routinely threw away the enclosed drug warnings before she (or I) could read them. Yet, Mom had every right to know what the drug warnings said. Obviously, she knew better than I about how they made her feel and whether they were helping or hindering her quality of life.

And then there were the routine procedures, both in and out of the hospital, that I rarely objected to. For example, when Mom started seeing our family doctor, he ordered her to have a mammogram. After her scan, she said to me, "Why do they make women my age go through this?" Now, I wholeheartedly agree with her. Would detection of breast cancer, a fundamentally slow growing disease, have benefited an eighty-five year old woman? The treatment itself would have probably killed her. (Luckily, mammograms are no longer routinely recommended for women after age seventy-five.)[10] Yet, this lack of understanding on the part of her physician made my role as Mom's health care proxy even more important. Let's investigate this topic further. . .

Prevent, Cure or Manage Disease?

Generally speaking, doctors are trained to *cure* disease, not prevent it. (After all, if doctors were good at prevention, our medical care system would not be overflowing!) But in many ways, doctors are not very good at curing either. More and more disease states are being classified as chronic conditions, where physicians feel they have no choice but to "manage" a disease rather than cure it. In Dr. Kathryn Collin's book *How Healthy is Your Doctor?*, she explains this approach in the field of traditional Western medicine:

> *"We're taught reactive medicine: we look for and find disease, then 'treat' what we find, alleviating the patient's symptoms and hopefully slowing their disease progression. Often, though, we're not impacting how or why the disease occurred in the first place, nor are we considering what might be done to prevent it from recurring."* [11]

Diagnostic tests, although touted as "prevention" by many health organizations, are at best "early detection" devices - they don't prevent anything. Thus, more and more patients are living with "detected" diseases and doctors are becoming more and more "symptom managers." Consequently, the physicians' tool kit has evolved into a laundry list of drugs and procedures that do not necessarily cure, but rather reduce pain and mask symptoms - along with expensive diagnostic tests that monitor the effects of these drugs and procedures.

Physicians mean well and sometimes their tactics are warranted. But it's important to be proactive and well-informed about any medical treatment. After all, when was the last time your loved one's doctor read aloud the warnings on a prescription before he or she handed it out? Or explained the potential interactions of the various drugs your loved one was taking? Could some of the health issues your loved one is experiencing actually be side effects of the very medications being prescribed to help them?

ADRS (Adverse Drug Reactions)

Q. Why are adverse drug reactions (ADRs) so dangerous for the elderly?

A. The elderly are especially prone to ADRs because:

-   they often take multiple prescriptions, making interactions always a possibility;

-   accuracy in taking the drugs "as directed" is a challenge due to memory or physical issues;

-   drugs are processed less efficiently in the body than in a younger person, so "normal" doses can build up in the blood, making side effects more likely.

An article in the *British Journal of Clinical Pharmacology* pointed out the high correlation between aged persons and the risk and incidence of ADRs in a hospital setting. These occurrences, referred to as "type A or dose related," were "predictable from the known pharmacology of the drug and therefore potentially avoidable." Notably, it goes on to say that the *combination* of more than one drug in the blood stream could potentially make the risk of an ADR even greater than from just the single drug itself.[12]

Q. What can we do to protect our loved one from an ADR?

A. The most important thing is to recognize that ADRs from prescribed medications do exist and the incidence is not rare. Take my advice and read carefully the information included with your loved one's prescriptions. Make sure ALL of their doctors are aware of every medication they are taking and that they have checked for interactions. And be vigilant. If you see a change in behavior or health status, it might not be due to the disease. It could be due to the cure.

Personally, I wish I had had the foresight to do ADR research when I was caring for Mom. Had I fully understood the risk of ADRs, I would have explored more natural alternatives or discontinued some of her meds. Perhaps certain side effects and even some of her disease symptoms could have been reduced, or even eliminated, the need for the drugs themselves.

Disclaimer! Many prescription medicines have warnings about the potential harm of abruptly discontinuing the medication. Make sure you consult with the prescribing physician about any changes you want to make to your loved one's medical routine.

 The "American Geriatrics Society Beers Criteria" is a report published periodically to guide physicians on the appropriate use of drugs for the elderly. Created by a panel of experts and based on extensive study of drug research, the purpose is to provide information regarding the "potential" inappropriateness of certain drugs, the potential for ADR's, and the possible need for adjusted dosages when these medications are prescribed for older adults. There is also now a section in the report on alternative medications or non-medication options. You or your doctor might find this report helpful. See it at **healthinaging.org**.

Q. Can Clostridium difficile (C. diff) be a real problem for the elderly?

A. Yes. C. diff is a medical condition whereby harmful bacteria grows unchecked in a person's bowel and stool.

According to the Arizona Healthcare-Associated Infections Program[13], the most common cause of C. diff is frequent or prolonged antibiotic use which can kill off the good bacteria in the gut as well as the bad, and cause sometimes serious symptoms such as:

- watery diarrhea

- stomach pain or tenderness

- fever, sometimes severe

These symptoms can last for days, weeks or even years and in rare instances may become life threatening. This harmful bacteria can also be spread from one patient to another in medical facilities by inadequate hygiene on the part of caregivers. Most at risk for C. diff are:

- the elderly, especially those in medical care facilities

- people with weakened immune systems

- patients with serious underlying health conditions like cancer, liver or kidney disease

Not all diarrhea symptoms are caused by C. diff, of course, but it is something to be aware of when considering antibiotic drugs for the elderly.

Q. What is Sundowning Syndrome and how does it affect the elderly?

A. The Mayo Clinic describes it as "a state of confusion at the end of the day and into the night."[14] It manifests in people in different ways or a combination of ways, the most common behaviors being restlessness, anxiety, confusion, aggression, pacing or wandering.

According to the clinic, "Sundowning isn't a disease." It is fairly common in people with some form of dementia, such as Alzheimer's disease or vascular dementia, but the exact cause is unknown.

In Mom's five-year health care journey, I noticed her increased tendency to get anxious or paranoid in the evening. At first, she would get up in the middle of the night and stay up for two hours, occasionally checking the lock on her front door, and then go back to bed. I dismissed this as due to the recent traumatic events in her life and assumed it would subside as things normalized.

Yet, as time went on, she stayed up longer and longer during the night, and eventually began having anxiety around the same time each day, shortly after dark. In one way, it reminded me of the "colic" that my son had when he was a baby. Like colic, it presented itself as an apparent discontent or anxiety whose cause couldn't be pinpointed and whose effects couldn't be soothed.

Q. How can Sundowning Syndrome be addressed without medications?

A. Certain things seem to affect the severity of the condition.
Too much stimulation at the end of the day; not enough indoor light (shadows seem to be a major source of worry); disruption or lack

of routine in sleeping patterns; and seasonal decrease in the hours of daylight. (Knowing this, it makes sense that older people tend to like the southern climes more than the northern ones, not only for its warmer temperatures but for the slightly longer daylight hours in the winter time.)

According to the Mayo Clinic, many times physicians try to relieve severe "sundowning" symptoms with anti-psychotic drugs. The clinic, however, suggests that there are often non-pharmaceutical therapies that can be tried first. These include:

+ limiting naps in the daytime

+ restricting caffeine and sugar intake to the morning

+ planning outside activities that increase sun exposure

If you have a loved one who is experiencing "sundowning" I encourage you to work with them to explore non-medical relief of their symptoms. Individuals suffering from this syndrome may also be more susceptible to hospital delirium when in a medical facility (see "Hospital Delirium", Lesson 5.)

Q. Are there legitimate alternatives to traditional Western medicine?

A. As mentioned in Lesson 2, some patients turn to Integrative Medicine practitioners who often use a variety of the alternative healing modalities. These treatments may take the form of:

+ dietary changes or food-based additions to the diet

+ improving daily habits such as increased water consumption

+ more exposure to sunlight

+ more frequent social interaction

+ changing habits such as quitting smoking, decreasing alcohol consumption or implementing daily exercise

+ enlisting therapies for stress reduction and sense of well-being such as massage, cognitive therapies, biofeedback, meditation

✚ incorporating non-traditional healing therapies such as Chinese medicine, homeopathy, naturopathy, acupuncture, aromatherapy, Ayurveda medicine or chiropractic

The internet is a useful resource to explore these alternatives. Simply type "Alternatives to (name the medical condition, medication or proposed treatment)" or "Natural alternatives to…" in the search box of your browser. However, be cautious that the information you glean is from reputable sites. And look for more than one source to verify the information.

Note: Most alternative treatments are not backed by scientific research (as such research is very expensive) and the lack of government regulation can result in poor quality control of certain supplements. Also, results from these treatments may take longer than traditional drugs and may vary.

 Always consult with the attending physician or pharmacist to verify that there are no possible interactions between the alternative treatments you are considering and the pharmaceuticals or other treatments being administered to your loved one.

Also, it's a good idea to keep on hand a list of the patient's current medications, especially if the person is transferred from one medical facility or medical unit to another. As much as we want to trust that medical records follow the patient wherever they go, the system is not seamless and omissions do occasionally occur.

Finally, be aware that if prescription medications are supplied in a medical facility, they are being paid for by the patient or their insurance coverage. The patient may be entitled to the remainder of those medications when they are discharged or transferred to another facility.

Aggressive vs. Non-Aggressive Care

Q. What is meant by "aggressive" medical care?

A. A physician can use whatever tools are at his or her disposal to detect, cure or manage a medical problem - regardless of how painful or debilitating it might be to the patient. Typically, when someone is under a doctor's care, the default approach to their care is "aggressive." If a patient is admitted to an emergency room, hospital or rehabilitation facility, aggressive care is also the default approach and often involves "invasive" treatments or procedures.

However, for the elderly, this may not be the best approach. As their health care proxy, we need to acknowledge this and to understand what constitutes "invasive" procedures and be vigilant about their implementation.

Q. What is an invasive medical procedure?

A. The National Cancer Institute defines it as "a medical procedure that invades (enters) the body, usually by cutting or puncturing the skin or by inserting instruments into the body." For an elderly person, this can be an important consideration because thinning skin and delicate veins make even minimally invasive procedures like needle insertion, for example, both difficult and painful. The skin bruises more easily and it does not heal as well, so infection is more likely.

According to the Mayo Clinic, a **"minimally invasive" procedure** is when "doctors use a variety of techniques to operate with less damage to the body than with open surgery." It often results in less pain, shorter hospital stays and fewer complications. Laparoscopic surgery, done through small incisions using small tubes and surgical instruments and with tiny cameras, is an example of this kind of surgery.

Q. What is a non-invasive medical procedure?

A. It would seem logical that this is a medical procedure that does not require any of the above. In other words, it is a conservative procedure that does not require cutting into the body or removing tissue. This definition can be expanded, however, to include no penetration of any body cavity beyond its natural opening. In that context, even a rectal examination would be considered invasive. So based on these definitions, a "non-invasive" procedure that does not enter the body would do no harm, right? Possibly, but possibly not. Let's look at one such "non-invasive" procedure - the body scan.

Physicians have numerous ways to look inside their patients in a non-invasive way, including x-rays (or CT scans), radioactive tracers (PET scans), radio waves (MRIs), and sound waves (ultrasounds), just to name a few. A report in *Radiology Research and Practice* indicated that sometimes frequent scans can carry the risk of over exposure to radiation, but there are two other down sides to consider as well.[15]

As mentioned earlier regarding Mom's mammogram, body scans often uncover abnormalities that are slow growing and are no immediate danger to one's health, or are a natural occurrence of aging. Yet, according to the same report, these test results can spawn more scans and occasionally, unnecessary biopsies and other invasive procedures. In other words, the more scans someone has, the more likely something abnormal will be found.

Q. Can there be negative psychological effects on the elderly from "non-invasive" procedures?

A. Yes. The mental and emotional stress of medical tests, including frequent doctor visits and unknown test results, coupled with sometimes increasing dementia, can be a recipe for acute or chronic anxiety or depression in the elderly.

In Chapter Four of the story, I explained how I would wait until the day of her appointment to tell Mom about it, because otherwise she would be up all night with worry. And in Chapter Ten, a hospital echocardiogram was attempted which ended up as an embarrassing incontinence episode for Mom and a failed attempt by the tech to get the scan. So elderly patients have more physical, mental and emotional limitations which make many procedures invasive, even if those procedures normally are not.

Additional fallout from all this, of course, is the increased participation required on the part of the caregiver or health care proxy to get the patient to the procedure or doctor's visit on time, to psychologically prepare them for the event, and to manage one's own worry and concern about the medical well-being of their loved one.

So, in retrospect, many of the treatments and procedures prescribed by physicians are often considered "invasive." In trying to align ourselves with the wishes of our loved one, it's important to understand the difference between an invasive and a non-invasive medical procedure and, with our understanding of the patient's health goals, support the limits on how far our loved one wants to go with a procedure.

Q. What constitutes a "routine" medical procedure?

A. These are procedures, invasive or not, which are done "routinely" to:

- provide baseline data needed for treatment

- to reduce liability on the part of the facility

- and/or to decrease the amount of time needed for hands-on care by the medical staff.

One thing is certain. The pain, inconvenience and/or expense of these "routine" practices are somehow passed on to the patient. The following medical procedures may be ordered for your loved one, especially when they are in a medical facility. Consider these options to see if they might be more in line with your loved one's health care goals:

❏ most medications administered by IV or PICC line can be stepped down and given orally instead [16]

❏ blood draws done for daily blood counts are often routine and can be refused [17]

❏ heparin injected on a daily basis to prevent blood clots may potentially be taken by mouth or substituted by other oral anti-coagulants [18]

❏ urinary catheterization can frequently be avoided if the patient can walk and use the bathroom or a bedpan [19]

❑ X-rays, CT and CAT scans can emit harmful radiation which Ultrasound, electrocardiogram (EKG), echocardiogram (ECG), or magnetic resonance imaging (MRI) do not. (Or recent scans might be obtained from other physicians, facilities instead of redoing the scan) [20]

❑ colonoscopy is not recommended after age seventy-five, however, a stool "guaiac" test is less invasive [21]

 You can locate the full article sources for each of the above items in the "Where I Got My Information" section of this book.

During her hospital stays, Mom was subjected to number of "routine" procedures that I learned later she might have avoided - with her protests (which she did) and my support of her wishes (which I often did not). Yet, on those rare occasions when I did object, the medical staff simply determined that those procedures weren't required after all. So it pays to speak up.

Before denying any procedure:

✔   ask what it is for

✔   determine if it's a routine policy

✔   and inquire what alternative (less invasive) method might be used

If you decide to deny or change the procedure, be sure that it is entered in your loved one's medical record, along with the reason. Remember, it is the facility staff's job to convince the patient that the procedures are necessary, but the patient reserves the right to refuse any treatment!

 Some hospitals now require doctors to sign off daily on "routine" procedures so the doctor knows that they are occurring.

Q. When you enter a hospital, is there a difference between "observation" versus "admission" status?

A. Yes. If the cost of the patient's hospital or subsequent rehab stay is considered "out-patient" services, it will often not be covered by "in-patient" insurance. In other words, those costs will become the patient's responsibility.

If your loved one experiences a medical problem outside of their primary care physician's office hours or if it's a situation that needs immediate attention, you will often be directed to go to the emergency room of your local hospital. There, the hospitalist might say he or she wants to keep the patient overnight for "observation", and you may have a tendency to automatically say "yes" - after all, what could it hurt?

Patients brought to the hospital emergency room are occasionally kept overnight for observation when they are not well enough to go home, but not sick enough to be formally admitted to the hospital for treatment. However, there is something the patient may not know under these circumstances. At this writing, in order to be covered by Medicare and/or their MAP insurance plan, the patient must be admitted to the hospital and remain there for three days, not including the day of discharge. [22]

A new federal law was scheduled to go into effect in 2016 called "The Notice Act," which would require hospitals to notify patients after twenty-four hours if they were still on "observation" rather than "admission" status, and to explain what that meant. There was also legislation introduced to Congress which would count observation days toward the three-day insurance requirement to cover the hospital or nursing home stay. So far, I have found no evidence that either of these laws have gone into effect. Perhaps you will have better luck in your research.

 On the United Hospital Fund website **nextstepincare.org/Caregiver_Home/Observation**, an article entitled "What is 'Observation Status'?" suggests that if your loved one is in that situation, you should ask whoever you come in contact with, "Has my family member been officially admitted to the hospital, or is he or she still under observation status?" and keep track of the responses and from whom until you get a satisfactory answer.

Q. When is it time to get a second opinion?

A. The answer is, whenever you feel it is necessary. Here are some
questions to guide you in that determination:

✔ How is the physician addressing the goal of your loved one in regard
to their health, and what is the goal of the treatment?

✔ How invasive is the treatment and what are the possible side effects?

✔ Can the patient carry out the treatment themselves or do they need help
for it to be effective?

If you are not satisfied with the physician's answers to these questions,
you may consider getting a second opinion and hearing another physician's
perspective about a prognosis or form of treatment.

 *For support, refer to "Shared Decision Making," Lesson 2; "Is
There Something Called Patient Rights?" Lesson 3; and "A Guided
Conversation," Lesson 1.*

If the second opinion is not an option or not satisfactory, there is one
additional recourse...

Q. What does it mean to be AMA (Against Medical Advice)?

**A. This is when a patient or their health care proxy goes against the
doctor's advice** and refuses a treatment or medical procedure or
admission to a healthcare facility. *The New York Times* cited a study in
The Journal of the American Geriatrics Society that analyzed a large
national sample from 2013 and found that "50,650 hospitalizations of
patients over age 65 ended with AMA discharges."

The article went on to say that hospital facilities may pressure patients
to sign an AMA form indicating that they are cognizant of their decision
to leave treatment. But this form is not actually required. Some physicians
even threaten patients that their health insurance will not cover their visit
if they leave. But this is false information. One concern of hospitals is
that those discharged against medical advice have higher rates of hospital
readmissions (which now trigger financial penalties for hospitals from
Medicare).[23]

Lesson 5: Be Ready For Rehab

As was mentioned in Chapter Four of the story, I was shocked when a hospital nurse told me that Mom needed to be sent to a rehabilitation facility. My only reference to what this meant was hearing about celebrities who had battled drug or alcohol addiction. Mom didn't have any such dependencies, and when she entered the hospital with a mild heart attack, she had been living somewhat independently and could walk, bathe, dress, brush her teeth, feed herself, have a conversation, do simple tasks and knew where she was. Seven days later, most of that was gone. What had happened?

You may remember my description of how the hospital's orders for Mom to remain in bed affected her. Looking back, it inflicted both mental and physical torture, and the decline in her quality of life during that short period of time was almost shocking. Within hours of her admission, she changed from an upbeat, kind and loving person to someone who was irrationally gripped by fear, suspicion, uncooperativeness and who seemed at times to be hallucinating. I knew the staff were overworked (they were not shy to talk about it when asked.) But because of this, there was little accommodation for someone with mental impairment who needed extra care. If I had not been there 24/7, most likely Mom would have survived on sleeping pills and anti-psychotic meds throughout her stay.

By day four in the hospital, Mom had stopped eating, become withdrawn and uncommunicative, and literally changed into a person I didn't know. It was indeed scary, and I felt helpless to soothe or to reason with her.

For the next three months, my husband and I cared for a person who not only had multiple medical problems, but had rapidly progressing dementia and undiagnosed delirium - and also needed extensive physical and occupational therapy. Let's take a closer look at this situation, the likelihood of it, and what, if anything, could have been done about it.

What is Deconditioning?

According to an article published by The National Institutes of Health,

> *"Deconditioning is a complex process of physiological change following a period of inactivity, bedrest or sedentary lifestyle. It results in functional losses in such areas as mental status, degree of continence (ability to pee on one's own) and ability to accomplish activities of daily living. It is frequently associated with hospitalization in the elderly." (In this situation) "muscle strength decreases by two to five percent per day" (and the loss of leg strength can lead to) "falls, functional decline, and increased frailty."* [24]

So deconditioning in hospitals can make patients weaker than they were when they were admitted, and inadvertently turn the hospitals into feeder institutions for rehab facilities where patients are sent to regain their strength (or some of it) that was lost while they were in the hospital. Brilliant.

Q. Are there other reasons that patients are sent from a hospital to rehab?

A. Yes. These include:

- a hospital's main focus is "acute" care to get the patient stabilized;

- most hospitals are at maximum capacity;

- hospital stays are generally more expensive for the patient than rehab care;

- Medicare and other health insurance programs have a limit of how many days they will cover expenses in a hospital setting.

Besides the likelihood of deconditioning, there is another serious reason to get patients up and out of the acute environment of a hospital… the **high risk of infection** that occurs from just being there. In fact, the U.S. Centers for Disease Control reports that on average 1 in 25 hospital patients suffer from a hospital-caused infection. And in 2011, an estimated 75,000 patients died of such infections during their hospitalizations.[25]

But just as important for the patient is the high instance of hospital delirium…

Q. How common is "hospital delirium"?

A. Quite common. The American Geriatrics Society notes that some of the physical conditions that can trigger delirium are [26]:

- infection (especially of the urinary tract)

- adverse reaction to medications

- hypoxia (the absence of enough oxygen for bodily functions)

- uncontrolled pain

- hypoglycemia (low blood sugar)

- electrolyte imbalance (tiny dietary compounds, usually salts, that are needed to transmit small electrical impulses for bodily functions.)

A study by Dr. Dennis Popeo published in the *Mt. Sinai Journal of Medicine* states that physicians often have difficulty identifying delirium and will misdiagnose it unless they take into account other predisposing conditions that make an elderly patient more susceptible, such as vision or hearing impairment, severe illness or cognitive issues. He goes on to provide shocking statistics about the incidence of hospital-induced delirium among the elderly [27]:

- 6–56% in general hospital admissions with "a higher prevalence associated with increased age and increased severity of medical illness"

- 32% in general intensive care unit

- 42% in cardiac intensive care units;

- 9–87% in post-operative units

To decrease such risk, Dr. Popeo says it's important to alter some hospital procedures. These include minimizing the use of physical restraints, bladder catheters and iatrogenic (doctor ordered) events, and to maintain appropriate nutrition for the patient. Other practices that can help ease episodes of delirium:

✚ frequent cognitive orientation

✚ decreasing environmental stimuli

✚ increasing mobility

✚ preventing dehydration

✚ monitoring medications

He notes that some physicians also turn to anti-psychotic drugs, but this should be a last resort, as such therapy has had controversial results. Taking steps to prevent delirium before it appears is the best approach.

A study published on hospital delirium in *JAMA Psychiatry* [28] underlines the high incidence of delirium among hospital patients over 70 years of age who already have dementia symptoms, and the likelihood of delirium worsening and hastening those dementia symptoms long-term.

Another delirium study published in *Worldviews on Evidence-Based Nursing* [29] states that medical professionals need to partner with family members and caregivers to watch for signs of delirium in order to quickly diagnose the problem and minimize its devastating effects on their loved ones. And in order to do that, it says, patient advocates need to know what to look for:

❏ problems with attention, concentration, memory, disorientation

❏ difficulty tracking conversations and following instructions

❏ thinking and speech disorganized, slow or rapid delivery

❏ quick-changing emotions, easy irritability, tearfulness

❏ new paranoid thoughts or delusions (i.e., fixed false beliefs)

❏ new perceptual disturbances (e.g., illusions, hallucinations)

❏ motor skill changes such as slowed or decreased movements

❏ restlessness

❏ wake cycle changes. i.e., asleep during day, awake at night

❏ decreased appetite

Encouragingly, the above study states that when caregivers and family members are educated about delirium, and work in partnership with the health care provider, the incidence of delirium drops and the stress on the caregivers and family may also subside. In summary, if your loved one is hospitalized or is in any medical facility and shows a marked and sudden negative change in behavior or personality, or has risk factors that could bring on delirium, notify the doctor immediately and insist on an evaluation or preventive measures for delirium.

Skilled Nursing Rehab

The rehabilitation required to regain (or partially regain) one's strength after a hospital stay can involve in-house therapies which typically occur in one of two places:

- a separate facility within the hospital called an "Inpatient Rehab" unit (IRF)

- or a "Skilled Nursing/Rehab" facility (SNF) or Skilled Nursing Unit (SNU) in a nursing home

The main thing to know is that when a patient is admitted to skilled nursing rehab, the person's medical insurance dictates what happens next. Since health insurance plans pay most of the costs of the patient's stay (see "Paying For Rehab", page 150) these insurance plans dictate strict rules that the rehab facility must follow.

Q. In a hospital rehab unit (IRF), what is expected of the patient?

A. The current Medicare and Medicaid rule states,

> *"The IRF medical record must demonstrate the patient is making functional improvements that are ongoing, sustainable, and of practical value, as measured against the patient's condition at the start of treatment."* [29]

What does this mean? Patients admitted to an IRF must be able to tolerate an intense regimen of therapy each day. In this scenario, the hospitalist has a "face-to-face" visit with the patient every few days to assess their progress and to review their therapy plan. If the rehab patient cannot tolerate an intense regimen of therapy, or has dementia or other chronic illness, or the hospital does not have its own rehabilitation unit, then the patient will most often be transferred to a nursing home or SNF for their rehabilitation. There is also an arrangement in some hospitals called "swing beds", where SNF beds are reserved in the acute patient wings if needed for skilled nursing rehab care.

Q. How does rehabilitation at a skilled nursing facility (SNF) differ from an IRF?

A. The website medicare.gov states that rehabilitation therapy in a SNF:

- includes physical therapy, occupational therapy and speech- language pathology

- patients are evaluated within twenty-four hours of arriving at the facility and therapy sessions usually begin shortly thereafter

- the amount of therapy time varies depending on the patient's health status and endurance, but it is typically 1.5 hours/day, most days of the week

- the patient is expected to actively participate and benefit from the program

- the physician is required to make a face-to-face visit with the patient at least once every thirty days to evaluate their physical (and mental) condition and modify treatment, if needed

This last point is important. It was my experience that you will not see the physician at an SNF much sooner than that. Most of these doctors are family physicians who take on multiple nursing homes for extra income, in addition to their own patient case load. For this reason, they may visit the rehab at odd or unpredictable times. And meeting the doctor for the first time, as we did, after your loved one has been in the facility for nearly thirty days, is not very supportive. However, this is when you can most effectively bring up concerns and ask questions.

So, it's important to check with the rehab staff to see when the doctor is expected or to get his office phone number and leave a message that you would like to talk with him or her, even if it's by phone. In the doctors' absence, there's usually a Physician's Assistant (PA) who is more hands on and communicates with the doctor about patient issues that arise in the rehab facility.

According to the American Academy of Physician Assistants, PAs are "nationally certified and state-licensed medical professionals who have the authority to examine, diagnose and treat disease." They are allowed to prescribe medications, interpret diagnostic tests and do medical procedures. But the PA is ultimately under the supervision of the board-certified physician. If you ever disagree or question the advice or direction of the PA, you can insist on speaking directly with the doctor. The PA may not like it, but don't let that deter you.

Therapists, nurses and nurses' aides make up the rest of the rehab medical team. As they make their "rounds" to visit each patient on a daily basis, don't hesitate to ask them questions or get feedback on your loved one's progress.

 Under special circumstances, such as an acute health issue, the rehab patient may be allowed to stay in the rehab facility during a brief break from therapy.

Q. What is the role of the social worker in a medical facility?

A. In most hospitals and skilled nursing rehab facilities, they are hired to interact with patients, especially on admission and once again at discharge. These persons can potentially be another layer of advocacy for your loved one in certain situations, so its important to confirm if there is a social worker on staff in the facility and if so, what their role and function is, as this can vary from place to place.

Learning the scope of the social worker's expertise and influence in these settings will also help you manage your expectations about how much help they can provide. To be honest, during the several times Mom was in medical facilities, I was probably expecting (and wishing for) a lot, as I didn't have anyone else to consult with. So my encounters with the hospital and rehab social workers did not seem very helpful. As much as they appeared to empathize with our situation, I felt their main priority was to encourage us to comply with the physician's orders. Perhaps my experience was an exception or perhaps my disappointment was partly due to not knowing what their actual role was. So let's explore the basics.

The National Association of Social Workers states that the role of the social worker in a medical institution can include:

-   helping patients and their families to understand illness and treatment options, as well as side effects and/or consequences of various treatments or treatment refusal;

-   educating patients on the levels of health care (e.g., acute, sub-acute, home care);

-   entitlements (patient rights);

-   community resources and advance directives;

-   facilitating decision making on behalf of patients and families;

-   coordinating patient discharge and continuity of care planning.

Some social workers leave the first task above to a "nurse manager" or "patient case manager," if there is one. Others specialize in Medicare and health insurance issues and Medicaid applications. It's best to ask the social worker what specific services he/she provides, so that your expectations do not fall beyond the scope of what they offer and so you can address your concerns to the right person, even if that person is the physician.

From my experience, hospital social workers will not be of much help if you need to choose a rehabilitation facility. Perhaps they are ethically bound to not make recommendations. However, they may be able to tell you if any recent complaints against a particular facility have been filed with local or state authorities.

Q. What are the benefits of a "care conference" or "rounding"?

A. This is when the clinical staff visits the patient's room to discuss with the patient and their family the patient's progress, treatment options and discharge plans. By law, a patient is allowed to participate in formulating their own hospital treatment and rehabilitation treatment plan (see "Shared Decision Making," Lesson 2) based on their health goals. So one thing that the social worker should be able to do, which I wasn't aware of during Mom's stays, was to arrange and facilitate a "care conference" - or in a short term stay it might be called a "rounding."

The experience of Mom's hospital and rehabilitation admissions left me feeling like a deer dazed in headlights. People came into her room and introduced themselves, but with Mom and I functioning on little sleep and this whole situation being new to us, it all seemed very disjointed. In fact, I was "warned" by Mom's physical therapist at the rehab facility that her "refusal" to cooperate with their plan could result in non-coverage by her insurance. If I had known that we could have a voice in deciding her treatment, perhaps things might have gone differently. I would have had the all important discussion about the fact that Mom wanted me with her during her therapy sessions, and that she needed twenty-four hour care while in rehab and what were our options?

To avoid this dilemma with your loved one, shortly after they are admitted to a hospital or rehab facility, you or your loved one should request a "care conference" or "rounding" through the facility's social worker. This meeting might include the social worker, nurse case manager or PA, health care proxy and/or family, the attending doctors (if its in a hospital) or therapists (if in a rehab facility) and the patient (if it will not cause them undo anxiety.) Here is when your loved one's health goals, current health status, therapy plan and discharge plan can be discussed, agreed upon and coordinated.

 If your loved one is being admitted for a permanent stay at a facility (see Lesson 7: Choose the Right Place For Your Loved One) these conferences are required by state law and take place within two weeks of residency and then once per quarter. They are not required for temporary stays, however, so your loved one or their advocate should insist on such a conference.

Paying for Rehab

Q. Who pays for rehab?

A. The most common answer is... a government and/or private medical insurance program. If your loved one is age sixty- five or older, this might be Medicare A, or more likely, a combination with a Medicare Advantage Plan (MAP) or other private health insurance.

The reason for MAP is that as medical costs escalate, even if Medicare pays for 80% of the rehab stay initially, the other 20% due can be quite a financial burden to the patient. So MAP or "gap" insurance has become the common solution, where private insurance plans pick up the difference between the health care costs and what Medicare A will pay - although deductibles and strict qualifying conditions still apply.

At this writing, Medicare, MAP or a private insurance plan can potentially pay for up to 100 days of a rehab stay, depending on the patient's progress with their therapy. Prior to 2013, patients in rehab needed to show "measurable improvement" over a specified period of time in order to have their therapy costs covered. However, in 2013, a new ruling in Medicare policy determined that if a patient's "functional abilities would deteriorate without these services" then what is called "maintenance therapy" could take place.

Maintenance therapy is not covered indefinitely, however, and with private insurance companies now driving the rules of payment, more and more notices of termination of coverage in nursing homes are being activated in as early as seven days after the patient arrives. If a notice is given, there is an appeal process (check with your rehab facility for details), but be aware that even as an appeal is granted, more notices may reoccur throughout the rehab stay.

Q. What is Medicaid and can it pay for rehab stays?

A. Medicaid, a combined federal and state run program, is currently only rarely being used for short-term rehab and skilled nursing home stays. It was originally devised to cover health care costs that Medicare would not, and eligibility was based on the patient's annual income and available assets. The patient's income had to be less than the cost of their medical care and there was (is) a monetary limit on the person's assets. Spousal assets and income were also a factor.

However, Medicaid's ability to pay these health care costs has declined so greatly in recent years, that many nursing homes have opted out of becoming certified to accept it. Each state has their own requirements for eligibility in Medicaid, and some people qualify for both Medicare and Medicaid. For more information, ask your rehabilitation facility social worker. There are also elder law attorneys in each state who specialize in Medicaid applications.

 Certain states also have a "Medicare Savings Program" that may help you save ahead for Medicare premiums, deductibles and coinsurance. For more information about this or Medicaid, contact your state's Medical Assistance Office.

Disclaimer! As of 2017, the political climate in the U.S. may alter Medicare and/or Medicaid as it is currently known. Please consult with your medical or legal experts for further advice!

 Medicare currently has a website at **medicare.gov/inpatientrehabilitationfacilitycompare/** that outlines:

• how Medicare pays for inpatient rehab stays;

• compares doctors, hospitals and in-patient rehab facilities;

- gives infection rates for these facilities;

- and lists providers and suppliers who are "at risk for termination from Medicare."

Lesson 6: Consider Bringing Them Home

If you've read Mom's story, you know that we initially moved her into a rehabilitation facility without knowing that there was an option to do her rehab at home. When we finally decided to move her out of the rehabilitation facility, strictly to get her (and us) out of that environment, we were surprised to learn that the treatments and therapies offered "in house" at the facility could come home with her.

Although some caretakers welcome the respite of having their loved ones receive their rehab therapies at a rehab facility, from my experience, if your loved one has moderate to severe dementia or hospital delirium, they will not receive the care and supervision they need in a hospital or other medical facility unless you are with them continuously or pay someone out-of-pocket to be there 24/7. Such patients are often considered a burden to the hospital staff, a fall-risk liability and assumed to be potentially uncooperative.

Either my husband or I had been "living" with Mom at her rehabilitation facility for several weeks, and we were anxious to leave and make it easier on ourselves. Yet, I had no idea of the totality of services to which Mom was entitled when we finally brought her home. And neither the rehab social worker, the home health care agency, the rehab facility doctor nor the home health care physician's assistant fully explained it to us. So we didn't take advantage of some of the additional home nursing care that came along with Mom's therapy program and could have given my husband and I a much needed respite. Let's take a closer look. . .

Medical Coverage for Home Rehabilitation

Here's a memorable quote from the U.S. Government Medicare website:

> *"Home health care is usually less expensive, more convenient, and just as effective as care you get in a hospital or skilled nursing facility."*

I would add to that fewer complications from infection, fewer drug errors and less hospital delirium! So let's see an overview of how Medicare A and Medicare Advantage Plans work in a home remedial care situation.

Q. How does one qualify for Medicare to pay or in-home rehabilitation services?

A. The person must have been in a hospital or in a rehabilitation facility, under the care of a doctor and hire a home health agency that is approved by Medicare. Also, the patient must be basically homebound and unable to leave the home without some kind of assistance. At the time of this writing, under these conditions, Medicare and MAP will pay for services provided by the home health agency which are specifically ordered by the doctor.

Q. What services are covered by Medicare for in-home rehabilitation?

A. Typically, this is what is covered:

✚ skilled nursing care

✚ physical, occupational and other therapies

✚ social services such as counseling

✚ medical supplies such as equipment (i.e., wheelchair), and wound supplies.

This is what *isn't* covered:

- 24-hour a day home care

- meals delivered to the home

- homemaker services like shopping, cleaning and laundry when this is the only care you need

- personal care like bathing, dressing, toileting, when this is the only care you need.

- also, 20% of the Medicare-approved amount for medical equipment is paid by the patient or their MAP insurance.

The above information was gathered from a document called "Medicare and Home Health Care" on the Medicare website **medicare.gov**. You are strongly advised to visit this website or call 1-800-MEDICARE (1-800-633-4227) to get the most up-to-date policy changes.

Q. How is the home health care plan for rehabilitation decided?

A. Home health care plans that will be covered by health insurance need to be initiated and approved by a doctor. Any change in care also requires a doctor's approval and in my experience, can sometimes be slow to implement because of the red tape involved. However, as with the skilled nursing care in a nursing home, most often a physician's assistant will do the doctor visits to the home and carry out the doctor's orders.

 As with the nursing home, if you do not agree with or you want to question the doctor's orders for treatment, you have the right to contact the doctor directly, regardless of the PA's insistence that they can relay the information.

Q. Does Medicare guarantee their home rehabilitation patients certain rights?

A. Yes. Medicare patients have certain rights and should expect a certain level of care. According to the Medicare website, these rights include:

✔ having the patient, their home and property treated with respect

✔ being told in advance of any care plans or changes to the plan

✔ rights to privacy

✔ appeal rights or how to file a complaint

✔ written confirmation of what the patient will be required to pay;

✔ involvement in care decisions

✔ training of caregivers on how to perform care

✔ quick response to changes in health or behavior

✔ quick response to patient requests

Q. Can a patient switch their in-home rehabilitation provider?

A. Yes, but once you "lock in" with an agency it can be a trying experience to switch providers. I encourage you to do your "due diligence" before signing a contract. And be aware that you are not obligated to use a provider that is recommended by a hospital, nursing home, or doctor.

How do we do our due diligence? In most U.S. cities, the home health care agency market is very competitive. Get all the details of what the agency will provide, as well as:

❑ What, if any, cost will be out of pocket to the patient

❑ Check their client references

❑ Inquire about their policies regarding contacting the attending physician directly

❑ What is their policy about referring to hospice care?

❑ What is their call back response if you have a question

❑ Typical turnover in staff, etc.?

Here is an online app that let's you compare different home health care agencies in your area - **medicare.gov/homehealth compare/**

Lesson 7: Choose the Right Place For Your Loved One

As described in Chapter Nine of the story, when my husband and I were taking care of Mom, we came to a point where we could no longer provide care 24-hours a day, nor could we afford a 24-hour companion. So I decided to look for an adequate living situation for her. The home care agency physician's assistant told us that he didn't think she needed a memory care arrangement (although we suspected otherwise.) So, with many different housing options available, finding the right place for Mom was a challenging task.

As you may remember also from the story, Mom ended up never moving to the place we finally found. Yet, the point is, if you have children and have ever experienced the agony of picking out an appropriate school for your child, you can imagine the even greater challenge of finding the right place for your aged loved one. To help with this task, below is a discussion of some of the choices that abound.

Long-Term Care Facilities

During a major health decline of a loved one or eventually in anyone's health journey, living independently or without help may no longer be an option. When this happens, especially if it appears suddenly, family members may step in, but the majority of your loved one's care will probably fall to one person. Whether it is you, as their health care proxy, or someone else, it is important to recognize that the situation with your loved one is now in a fluid state and will not remain the same over time. If anything, it will become more demanding.

At some point, the medical needs of the loved one will go beyond the skills of the caregiver; or the patient may experience serious dementia symptoms that make it unsafe for them to continue living in a home setting; or perhaps the caregiver will experience burnout (see Lesson 9: Remember, It's Not Your Journey.) So as your loved one's health care proxy, it's important that you gather your support team (whoever that might be) and address these concerns before problems arise:

❏ What are the wishes of your loved one regarding their health?

❏ Who will provide their care and where?

❏ How will their medical needs be managed?

❏ Can the caregiver sufficiently carry out the treatment or do they need help?

❏ How will the care be paid for?

❏ Will the health (both mental and physical) of the caregiver be protected?

❏ If the need for care changes, what will be the next step?

Each person's situation and needs are different. Part of the health care proxy's responsibility is to work with and assess those needs. If the guided conversation mentioned in Lesson 1 has taken place, the solution may be more easily determined. If it hasn't, the situation may come up unexpectedly and be problematic for both the family and the patient.

Moving your loved one to a long-term, live-in facility can bring peace of mind that their basic needs are taken care of and the family can visit them and have a life of their own. Some elderly people are very social and thrive in such a group environment. Others will have nothing to do with it. Either way, it's important to recognize that the care provided in a health institution is not the necessarily the same quality and certainly not the same frequency as home care. These places are, for the most part, understaffed and overwhelmed.

If the patient needs a lot of care and attention, generally speaking they won't get it unless you or another advocate of your loved one are there to make sure it happens or pays for private duty care at the facility. This can be out of the realm of possibility for the typical family, so many times we move our loved one to a long-term care facility and just hope for the best.

On Medicare.gov, there's an app called "Nursing Home Compare" that ranks various facilities in your area based on federal inspection reports. This does not take the place of actually visiting the facility, of course, but it does provide a starting point if there are several places to choose from.

Q. What types of long-term care facilities are there?

A. There are basically five types on the market in the U.S. at the time of this writing. They are:

- Continuing Care Retirement Communities (CCRC)

- Assisted Living Facilities

- Residential Care Homes (Adult Family Homes, Board and Care Homes, Small Group Homes)

- Nursing Homes or Skilled Nursing Facilities (SNF)

- Alzheimer Special Care Units (Memory Care Units or SCUs)

Q. What is the function of the Continuing Care Retirement Community (CCRC)?

A. These offer more than one kind of housing and different levels of care. Residents move from one level to another based on their needs, but usually stay within the CCRC. Most offer independent living in a housing development or apartment building as the first level of care. Some CCRC's will only admit people into their nursing home if they've previously lived in another section of their community, like assisted living or an independent area.

 If you're considering a CCRC, be sure to check the quality of the skilled nursing, rehab and memory care units as well. Your CCRC contract usually requires you to use the CCRC's nursing home if your loved one eventually needs nursing home care.

Q. What is offered at an Assisted Living Facility?

A. Residents often live in their own room or apartment within a building or group of buildings and have some or all of their meals together. Social and recreational activities are usually provided and some facilities offer health services on site. These facilities provide help with some activities of daily living and some help with personal care like taking medicine or getting to appointments.

☞ *Not all assisted living facilities provide the same services. In most cases, assisted living residents pay a regular monthly rent, and then pay additional fees for any services they receive. As with CCRCs, you may want to check out their rehab, nursing and memory care units for future reference.*

Q. How do Nursing Homes or Skilled Nursing Facilities differ from the above?

A. According to the National Institutes of Health, a nursing home is "a place for people who don't need to be in a hospital but can't be cared for at home... Some are even set up like a hospital." These patients often need 24-hour care, so most of these facilities have nurses' aides and skilled nurses on hand at all times. The staff can provide:

- rehabilitation therapy on a short-term basis;

- regular nursing care for very sick patients;

- assistance with daily activities like eating, dressing, bathing, medications, and walking;

- some facilities have special units for memory care.

Q. What is provided at Residential Care Homes?

A. Often a single-family dwelling in neighborhoods, residential care homes provide non-medical care for the elderly. Housing two to ten patients, they offer assisted living in a more home-like setting; private or shared rooms; meals; and help with medications and personal hygiene, housekeeping and transportation. Residents are often memory impaired or Alzheimer's patients.

 This model is relatively new in elderly care and may not be available in all cities. More information can be found at **aplaceformom.com/senior-care-resources/residential-care-homes**

Q. What can we expect from Alzheimer Special Care facilities or in-house Memory Care Units?

A. There are a few specialized nursing care facilities that serve only dementia patients and provide several levels of memory care. However, due to the increased occurrence of dementia in older patients, many long-term care facilities now offer separate living quarters dedicated solely to memory care. These units may be in 24-hour lock-down, depending on the severity of the patient's dementia, to prevent wandering.

 From my limited experience of dedicated Alzheimer facilities, they appear to provide a broader spectrum of programs and treatment options, and the staff is exposed to more high-level training to work with dementia patients.

Q. How much does long-term care cost?

A. According to the U.S. government website longtermcare.gov the average cost for a semi-private room in a nursing home in 2010 was $205 per day or $6,235 per month. For a private room, it was $229 per day or $6,965 per month. And a one-bedroom apartment in an assisted living facility was $3,293 per month. It's safe to say that these costs have risen significantly in recent years.

Q. Does Medicare cover long-term care?

A. Neither Medicare nor most private health care policies cover long-term care. As we have seen, Medicare A (hospital insurance) only covers some of the skilled nursing facility or rehab expenses after hospitalization for an acute illness or injury. It never covers other services in an assisted living or long-term residence. The few government subsidies that will cover senior care housing are financially restrictive and apply only to lower income groups.

Regarding Medicaid, what we learned in Lesson 5 basically holds true for long-term care. **LongTermCare.gov** makes it clear that getting coverage via Medicaid is not easy. "Medicaid does pay for the largest share of long-term care services for some patients, but to qualify, your income and assets must be below a certain level and you must meet minimum state eligibility requirements."

There are two other limited government long-term care programs, The Older Americans Act and certain benefits under the Department of Veterans Affairs, but they have even stricter rules than Medicaid. And of course, all of these offerings may change at any time.

So based on this information, it's clear that covering the cost of appropriate housing for our elderly is a huge issue. Unless they (and we) plan ahead - way ahead - the cost may outstrip the ability to pay. For this reason, people are turning to other ways to ensure their housing future.

Q. What is long-term care insurance and does it work?

A. It became popular in the 1980s and 90s and was intended to cover the cost of assisted living or in-home professional care toward the end of one's life. Problems began when insureds finally reached the age where they needed it, and long-term care costs had skyrocketed to the point where the premiums no longer covered all the expenses.

An article in the *Wall Street Journal* entitled "Long Term Care Insurance: Is it Worth it?" put it this way:

> *"People used to buy long-term-care insurance because they were scared. Now it is the policies themselves that are keeping buyers awake at night...The coverage has been coming under fire. Premiums have been rising, fewer insurers are selling the product, and new research is questioning whether many people even need it."* [30]

Recent attempts to rectify the short-comings of long-term care insurance policies are creating new financial vehicles. We'll take a brief look at some of them. More restrictions may apply. All have drawbacks as well as advantages.

Q. Are there new life insurance options?

A. Yes, there are four at present (with more to come I'm sure):

- *long-term care insurance combined with a life insurance policy* that pays out before you die for long-term care;

- *accelerated death benefits* that provides a tax-free advance on a life insurance policy for those with terminal illnesses;

- *life settlements* where you sell your life insurance policy for cash;

- and *vatical settlements* where a company buys your life insurance policy, pays the premiums, and pays out a percentage to you.

Q. What is an annuity and how does it pay for long-term care?

A. There are two. They are:

- *immediate annuity* where a person makes a single payment to an insurance company and they send back a guaranteed monthly amount

- and *deferred annuity* available to those under 65, where you make a single payment in exchange for monthly payments for long-term care and a deferred cash fund.

Q. Can reverse mortgages help pay for long-term care?

A. Possibly. There is one type available at present: *a home equity loan* that pays you cash for the value of your home without selling it. You must:

- be at least 62 years of age

- live in the home

- and meet with an approved reverse mortgage specialist.

   Disclaimer! For your protection, always consult with your financial advisor before purchasing or investing in any financial program.

The above financial information was taken from the **LongTermCare.gov** website

Q. What is the life expectancy in long-term care facilities (LTCFs)?

A. The U.S. Centers for Disease Control and Prevention website at cdc.gov/longtermcare estimates that over five million Americans are living in some kind of nursing care arrangement and:

- 1 to 3 million serious infections occur every year in these facilities;

- including urinary tract infections, diarrheal diseases and antibiotic resistant staph infections, to name a few;

- and infections are a major cause of hospitalization and death, with as many as 380,000 people dying from infections in LTCFs every year.

Results of a data-aggregate study in *BMC Health Services Research* showed similar results and concluded,

> *"The mortality rate showed that more than 50% died within 3 years, and almost a third of the residents may have needed palliative care within a year of admission. Considering the short survival time from admission, it seems relevant that (nursing) staff is trained in providing palliative care as much as restorative care."* [31]

(We will discuss palliative care in Lesson 8: Know When Enough Is Enough.)

These statistics can be interpreted in one of two ways. Either due to the high cost of being in a long-term care facility, many people opt to not be admitted until they are far past their ability to respond well in a institutional setting. Or, as was mentioned earlier, the care provided in long-term care settings does not meet the quality of home care, and the risk of infection from the facility itself is high. Either way, the results are telling.

For this reason, health care proxies and caregivers must be especially vigilant to notice unusual swings in mood or behavior, or sudden loss of appetite or reduced functionality that could be a sign of some kind of infection in our long-term care loved one.

If you do notice something, and you are acting as the health care proxy, then you need to decide if medical intervention (i.e., antibiotics, IV therapy or by mouth) is aligned with your loved one's goals for their health and end of life care.

There's No Place Like Home

Q. What is meant by "aging in place"?

A. "Aging in Place" is a major trend among the elderly today and refers to a person's desire to continue living in their own home as they age, rather than moving to an assisted living or other institutional arrangement.

Surprisingly, a large study done on aging adults by *The Gerontologist* and published in the *Oxford Journal* revealed that the preference to "age in place" had little to do with the dwelling itself. It seems that social connections to friends, neighbors, familiar places and knowing the location of local services made them feel safer in their homes and had the most positive impact. Interestingly, crime rate, housing conditions or other factors of the surrounding neighborhood, no matter how unsavory, did not play a role in disenchanting the aging home dweller. [32]

In order for the elderly to stay in their homes, several industries have sprung up to accommodate their needs. Companies provide physical adaptations to the home such as wheelchair ramps, bathroom grab bars, and raised toilet seats. Local senior services continue to expand their services in transportation, hot meals (even specialty meals for diabetics) and companionship. With the advent of self driving cars and grocery shopping online, as well as the recent push for walkable neighborhoods and telecommuting, the possibilities are expanding for aging in place.

 A word of caution: For some aging patients, their fervent wish is that you do whatever it takes to keep them at home. At times, the personal sacrifice required on the part of the caregiver to make this a reality is beyond one's capability. In Lesson 9, we will consider some parting thoughts on the subject of stress as it relates to caregivers and health care proxies. But one option to look at first is private duty home care.

Q. How does private duty home care work and is it affordable?

A. This is when a nurse aide or home care worker comes into the home for specified hours at a time, a few times a week (or more as needed) to relieve the primary caregivers and provide necessary support in hygiene tasks, household chores and companionship to the patient.

The website **medicare.gov** estimates that the average cost of an in-home nurse's aid is $21 per hour. I believe this estimate is typically low. It is also paid out of pocket by the patient and the cost varies depending on location, time of day, frequency, and tasks required. Evenings, weekends and holidays are usually more expensive. Extra charges may be incurred for services beyond basic services provided at nursing facilities.

Q. How does one hire a private duty home care worker?

A. There are two ways to hire a private duty home care aide - through an agency or independently. Both have advantages and drawbacks:

- If an aide is hired independently, usually the rate per hour is less. However, it will be necessary to publicize for applicants, interview them, do background checks and pay the employment taxes.

- If a hiring agency is used, you will pay a higher rate because of their services, but they will do all of the above for you. An important point is to make sure whomever you hire is licensed and bonded.

Q. Suppose you can't afford 24-hour private duty care?

A. Then another option is to look at what hours of the day are most critical to have a health care aide. Perhaps it is at night, or during meal times or in preparation for bed. For some loved ones, having help three hours during the day and three hours at night is enough to keep them living independently.

Whether you decide on a caregiver agency or an independent aide, it's important to do your due diligence by getting references! Also, you may want to secure a locked room in the dwelling where your loved ones valuables can be stored out of the way and out of sight, as an extra precaution.

 aarp.org/home-family/caregiving/planning-and-resources/ is one resource that has a search feature on their website where you can choose "Home Health Care Providers" and add a zip code to find home health agencies that serve your area.

Lesson 8: Know When Enough Is Enough

Anyone who has watched someone they care about go through medical procedure after medical procedure probably asks themselves at some point, is this worth it? There is hope that the person will progress and benefit from the medical intervention, but sometimes these procedures inflict more pain and suffering than the original problem itself.

This is especially true for the elderly. Considering the potential lifespan of the person, is prolonged treatment for a cure really what we are going for here? Or is it more important that they be able to live with dignity and perhaps in relative comfort with their malady or maladies and not be subjected to the unending invasive and intrusive aggressive care of a hospital or medical facility?

As you read in Mom's story, during her several hospital and rehab stays, I could see that her health was clearly deteriorating and I requested a hospice evaluation several times from her different doctors. However, I failed to get a recommendation from them and I lacked an understanding about the important role that her health insurance plan played in dictating the kind of medical treatment she was eligible for.

Although one doctor did eventually put Mom on "palliative care," during her second stay in the hospital, I must admit I did not witness any benefits from this. I don't know if I just was not aware of them or if this doctor's order did not really change the care that she was given.

So if I could do it all over again, I would request a second opinion directly from a hospice agency or find a doctor I could work with and/or ask what specific documentation and/or diagnostic tests were needed to qualify Mom for hospice under her health insurance plan. I now know how important it is for the health care proxy to understand what palliative care and hospice care are and to be ready to have it activated if their loved one needs it. Hopefully, this lesson will inform you as well.

What is Palliative Care and Hospice?

In Lesson 4, we learned that when our loved one enters the medical care system, the default approach of the physician and/or hospital facility is to implement an "aggressive" treatment plan. That is, to use whatever tools are at his or her disposal to relieve or cure the problem - no matter how painful or debilitating the treatment might be to the patient. At some point, the health care proxy may find themselves examining their loved one's treatment plan and questioning the appropriateness of this aggressive approach.

Thankfully, aggressive treatment is not the only course that a doctor can take, depending on a patient's health status. There are two other potential avenues physicians and hospitals may offer, whereby medical treatments can be looked at from a more holistic perspective. Depending on a patient's health status, their care can be directed as "palliative" or "hospice." As a health care proxy and voice for your loved one, you need to know what these are and the difference between them. Let's investigate each.

Q. Explain palliative care.

A. Palliativedoctors.org states that palliative ("pal-ee-uh-tiv") care is "for people who are seriously ill…whether that illness is curable, chronic or life-threatening." It provides:

✚ relief from pain and other uncomfortable symptoms

✚ assistance in making difficult medical decisions

✚ help with navigating the complexities of our health care system

✚ guidance in making a plan for care based on the patient's needs, goals and concerns

✚ emotional support

Physicians can be specially trained in this type of care and then lead a team of nurses, social workers, and other medical professionals to coordinate the care.

Palliative care initially gained some momentum in the late 1960's. By 2005, 25% of U.S. hospitals supported the program. Today, over 75% of U.S. medical facilities offer it.[33] However, if you are interested in this approach to care, it's important to check with the doctor and/or medical facility to make sure they offer it.

Sounds like something that should be made available for every seriously ill patient's medical care, doesn't it? If you accept palliative care as an option, I suggest that you get a detailed explanation of what changes in care will occur and make sure that they are carried out - because your loved one's insurance plan or their deductible will be paying for it.

Q. How does the purpose of hospice differ from palliative care?

A. Hospice is a subset of palliative care. The National Hospice and Palliative Care Organization describes the purpose of hospice care as:

✚ to manage pain and symptoms;

✚ address the emotional aspects of dying;

✚ supply needed drugs (to relieve nausea, pain, shortness of breath, agitation, etc.), medical supplies and equipment (i.e., hospital bed, wheelchair);

✚ guide the family regarding patient care (teach how to give injections, change dressings, etc.);

✚ provide respite for the caregiver when needed (volunteers offering companionship);

✚ bereavement counseling to surviving family and friends (for up to one year after the patient's death)

Q. How is hospice care carried out?

A. According to the above organization:

✔ All medical treatment for the condition shifts from cure to comfort.

✔ It's essentially end-of-life care, therefore hospice requires a "terminal" diagnosis.

✔ Hospice may be suggested by a health professional, but if not, the patient, family members or health proxy can initiate the conversation.

✔ As in palliative care, a doctor's order is required for hospice. If the patient's doctor or the hospice program itself does not agree with the eligibility of the patient, the patient or their health proxy can seek a second opinion.

Q. How will you know when to request hospice?

A. Like a "care conference" for those who enter rehab, you or the patient can request a "hospice consult" whenever you wish to discuss hospice. During the end stage of many diseases, a patient will often show weight loss, increased confusion, repeated infections, sometimes increased depression and sometimes increased lethargy. This used to be called 'failure to thrive' or 'end stage dementia' if it was dementia related. (Hospice intake staff now use a more "Medicare" friendly diagnosis.)

Q. How is a hospice consult arranged?

A. The health care facility's social worker is a good point person to arrange this with the doctor, the nurse or case manager, the health care proxy and/or family members and the patient (if this will not cause them undo anxiety or stress.)

It's important to get accurate information at the conference. For instance, although the physician's assistant at Mom's rehabilitation facility told me I needed two doctors to agree for a hospice diagnosis, this was incorrect. Only one doctor is needed. But you do need a doctor's order for hospice.

Q. Who pays for hospice?

A. In general, hospice is a qualified expense under Medicare A, MAP or Medicaid for people who likely have six months or less to live, based on their current prognosis. In most cases, the patient needs to be without effective treatment options, or with treatment options whose potential pain and suffering outweigh the possible benefits.

Typically, if a person is eligible for hospice, Medicare, Medicaid or other medical insurance will generally cover it 100%. There is no deductible and no copayment. Not only are the services of the hospice staff entirely covered, but medical supplies and prescriptions relating to pain and comfort management are also covered. This includes hospice services provided in a medical facility or provided in the home.

Q. What are the guidelines for hospice eligibility under Medicare and Medicaid programs?

A. According to a thesis entitled "Evaluation of the Prognostic Criteria for Medicare Hospice Eligibility," [34] here are the criteria *currently* used to qualify someone for hospice care:

-   The patient's condition is life-limiting

-   The patient and/or family have elected palliative treatment goals

-   The patient shows symptoms of severe physical debility (includes multiple emergency room visits or recent decline in functional status or 10% unintentional weight loss over the prior six months)

-   The patient shows signs of progression in disease severity (clinical or objective data obtained through serial physician assessment, or laboratory, radiologic or other studies.)

Since so much of the cost of hospice is covered by these health insurance programs, those entities determine the guidelines of when and how a person becomes eligible for hospice. This can be a frustrating experience for a health care proxy who clearly sees that their loved one is suffering and not benefiting from aggressive care, and yet, the patient or the proxy cannot get the doctor to agree to hospice due to an unclear prognosis.

Q. How does an unclear prognosis affect a doctor agreeing to hospice?

A. The thesis above proposes that Medicare's stringent criteria has lowered the incidence of long-term (months) stays in hospice for non-cancer patients over the last decade, at the same time that short-term hospice stays (days) have skyrocketed. It explores the disparity of when patients with cancer and those with non-cancer diagnoses (such as dementia or congestive heart failure) are deemed hospice eligible.

The erratic progression of this second category of illnesses present "plateaus of stability" at times (as in Mom's case) as compared to the gradual and often predictable decline of a cancer diagnosis. Therefore, the Medicare criteria for hospice can make it difficult for physicians to agree on the timing of this second group's eligibility - until it is sometimes too late to do much good. As a consequence, there is more caregiver burnout, less quality time for the patient spent in hospice care, and ultimately, more expense to the patient for acute hospital care.

An article entitled "Hospice Care Helps, But Often Doctors Don't Recommend It Soon Enough" in Harvard Health Publications of Harvard Medical School had this to say:

> *"Hospice care is underused...often because doctors don't suggest hospice to patients or delay referring them until shortly before death...referring a patient to hospice can seem like a sign of medical failure on their part. Many say they don't want to take away a patient's hope... hospice experts agree that most terminally ill patients benefit from being in hospice for at least three months before death."* [34]

Q. What can you expect from a Hospice Program?

A. According to "Next Step In Care", a program of The United Hospital Fund, in most cases hospice provides services in the patient's home or their residential living facility until the last few days before death, at which time there may be an option to move to a separate hospice facility. Here is how their services are arranged:

✚ In the home, once hospice is approved, a consultation is set up with a hospice nurse to explain the services the patient is entitled to, and to set up a schedule of care.

✚ Hospice workers replace other home nursing services which the patient may currently be receiving under Medicare. (For this reason, home care agencies and their attending physicians may appear reluctant to acquiesce their services to hospice care.)

✚ Most of the burden of patient care usually goes to the patient's family. A hospice nurse should be on call by phone 24-hours a day and can instruct the family on what to do in a medical emergency (stay at home, admit to a hospital, etc.)

✚ Hospice caregiver time not covered by Medicare can be supplemented with professional home care providers, but the patient pays for this out of pocket.

Not all hospice care programs are created equal, however, so you must do your due diligence. Here are some questions to ask when selecting a hospice program (taken from **nextstepincare.org**):

Disclaimer! All of the above information was accurate at the time of this writing. Please connect with your health care insurer for the latest information on hospice coverage.

❏ Is the hospice certified by Medicare?

❏ Is the hospice available by phone 24-hours a day?

❏ Will I have a nurse or case manager assigned?

❏ How does the hospice handle medical emergencies like difficulty breathing or severe pain?

❏ How much and what kind of equipment will the hospice provide?

❏ What are the hospice policies about giving pain medication, antibiotics, chemotherapy to relieve symptoms, radiation therapy, anti-nausea medication, blood transfusions, using mechanical ventilator support (breathing tubes), taking out implanted heart devices (pacemakers)?

A patient is regularly evaluated during a hospice program. If a patient's prognosis improves, or they show "stability" in their health status, their insurance program may "disqualify" or "graduate" the patient from hospice and no longer cover their hospice expenses. Also, your loved one or their health care proxy have the right to decline hospice care at any time and restart it later if necessary.

 A listing of hospice services available in your area can be found at **hospicedirectory.org.**

Lesson 9: Remember, It's Not Your Journey

As you have read in the story portion of this book, my journey as Mom's caregiver spanned five years. During that time, her needs steadily increased and I took on a larger and larger role in her care.

Toward the end of the five year period, my care was daily and then eventually hourly, until I started to experience caregiver burnout. At the very end, I felt guilt, exhaustion, depression, anxiety and emotionally numb. I experienced memory problems, sleep deprivation, migraines, toothaches, muscle tension and I gained twenty pounds.

What I experienced are just some of the possible symptoms of "caregiver stress syndrome". If we, as a caregiver or health care proxy, can be educated to recognize the existence and danger signs of this syndrome, perhaps we can not only avoid the unneeded consequences, but allow this critical time in our loved one's journey to be memorable in the most joyous sense. Let's learn more. . .

Caregiver Stress Syndrome

An article by the American Association of Nurse Anesthetists (AANA) entitled, "Understanding Caregiver Stress Syndrome," [36] enumerates these statistics on caregiving:

-   Each year, more than 44 million Americans provide unpaid care to an elderly or disabled person 18 years or older

-   Thirteen percent of caregivers are themselves elderly

-   Sixty- one percent of caregivers are women

-   Fifty-nine percent of unpaid caregivers have jobs outside the home

Q. What are the consequences of Caregiver Stress Syndrome?

A. According to the AANA, "Studies found that the physical symptoms of caregiver stress are a result of a prolonged and elevated level of stress hormones circulating in the body," possibly leading to:

1. increased risk for health problems, including high blood pressure, diabetes, and a compromised immune system

2. stress hormone levels like those suffering from *post-traumatic stress disorder*

This second consequence is very telling, wouldn't you say? The article goes on to explain, "The stress is not only related to the daunting work of caregiving but also the grief associated with the decline in the health of their loved ones."

So if you are experiencing caregiver stress syndrome, it is not your imagination. It is not your fault. And it does not make you a bad person. But what this syndrome can do, especially if you are the caregiver and the health care proxy, is cloud your judgment when it is needed most, keep you from hearing what your loved one wants and not allow you to enjoy those precious times of loving and caring for them, when it is much needed. So it's important to get help.

Parting Thoughts

Here are a few of my final thoughts on being a health care proxy:

> ✔ Our health care system best serves those who are resilient enough to tolerate and benefit from aggressive care and who do not suffer from the added medical complication of dementia. As the Baby Boomer generation ages and more and more people enter the system, it will fall upon the shoulders of the health care proxies to bridge that gap of customizing the health care system to fit their loved ones' needs. Accepting the responsibility as a health care proxy should never be taken lightly. Be sure you are informed and do your homework.

✔ Our job as a health care proxy is not to judge what they want, but to get what they want. To do this we have to *listen*. As you have read, I didn't know what Mom wanted because we never talked about it. Even so, when she was in the throws of her health crisis and mental impairment, I still could have listened. It is never too late. Don't make my mistake.

✔ Try journaling! Many of the notes for this book came from a journal I kept during Mom's health care journey. Journaling was not only a good way to document the progress or regression of her symptoms, which was helpful for doctor visits, for example, but it gave me a chance to quietly vent and then gain perspective on what was occurring. I highly recommend that you do the same. And it will be something you look back on and learn from later as well.

✔ I encourage you to identify helpful resources *before* your loved one is in a health crisis! In Mom's case, I was attempting to navigate the health care system with someone who had dementia. This added an extra layer of complication to an already challenging situation. I sought out caregiver information and support through the Alzheimer's Association, programs at memory care centers and a weekly support group at a nearby retirement center. See further resources below.

✔ Health crises often happen suddenly, or in the middle of the night. In those situations, it's easy to give in to the advice of the health care provider and just hope for the best. But that is not being an advocate for your loved one. To be the best you can be for them, be aware of when you are not thinking clearly or when you need more time to consider or discuss options. Find ways to take a break long enough to regroup before making a major decision. The attending physician can wait.

✔ Don't know what a procedure entails or the purpose of a medication or its side effects? Ask! The doctor or nurse may be miffed at your concern, but that's their problem. You are legally bound as a health care proxy for your loved one to find out - and that's the priority.

✔ You are not being neglectful if you refuse a treatment or admission to a facility because your loved one does not want it. From the health care worker's perspective, they have their reasons for wanting to do something. You have your reasons too. It's uncanny how some health care workers can make you feel guilty or even criminally negligent for going against what a doctor is recommending. Nevertheless, if you or your loved one don't want them to do something, JUST SAY NO! They will either not do it or if they are doing it, they will stop.

✔ To minimize the trauma to your loved one, especially if hospital delirium or dementia symptoms are suspected, request that any major procedures, transport, room changes, etc., be done during the day, whenever humanly possible. And, in my experience, perhaps avoid teaching hospitals for frail patients. These are institutions where student doctors and nurses learn their craft, which is admirable, but they may not be as experienced in working with the elderly population, plus the loved one may subjected to additional medical examinations and personnel.

✔ They will go how they will go. As much as we try to orchestrate the end of life care of our loved one, so much is out of our control. When they finally go, it will be on their terms, with the people they want to be there - if they want anyone. So NO GUILT!

✔ This final tip is based strictly on anecdotal evidence, but I have observed that families who have a medical professional in their ranks - whether it be a physician, nurse or someone else who knows the medical system and how it works - can potentially be influential in securing better care for their loved one. If you have that resource, I encourage you to introduce them to your loved one's doctors and nurses and let them know that this person will be consulting with you on your loved one's care. It might help.

The website **womenshealth.gov**, with the U.S. Department of Health and Human Services, is just one resource that offers good information about caregiver syndrome under the topic of "Caregiver Stress."

The National Council on Aging at **ncoa.org** is a good resource for caregivers and health care proxies. Or search "agencies on aging in (your town)" for local resources on the internet. The Rosalynn Carter Institute for Caregiving at **rosalynncarter.org** is also a notable resource. And of course, it's important to mention any caregiving stress symptoms to your doctor.

 To help you in your further research, see "Where I Got My Information" and other resources in the "Helpful Resources" section of this book.

"Helpful

Resources"

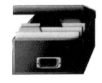

State of Ohio
Living Will Declaration
Notice to Declarant

The purpose of this Living Will Declaration is to document your wish that life-sustaining treatment, including artificially or technologically supplied nutrition and hydration, be withheld or withdrawn if you are unable to make informed medical decisions <u>and</u> are in a terminal condition or in a permanently unconscious state. This Living Will Declaration does not affect the responsibility of health care personnel to provide comfort care to you. Comfort care means any measure taken to diminish pain or discomfort, but not to postpone death.

If you would <u>not</u> choose to limit any or all forms of life-sustaining treatment, including CPR, you have the legal right to so choose and may wish to state your medical treatment preferences in writing in a different document.

Under Ohio law, a Living Will Declaration is applicable **only to individuals in a terminal condition or a permanently unconscious state**. If you wish to direct medical treatment in other circumstances, you should prepare a Health Care Power of Attorney. If you are in a terminal condition or a permanently unconscious state, this Living Will Declaration takes precedence over a Health Care Power of Attorney.

[You should consider completing a new Living Will Declaration if your medical condition changes or if you later decide to complete a Health Care Power of Attorney. If you have both a Living Will Declaration and a Health Care Power of Attorney, you should keep copies of these documents together. Bring your document(s) with you whenever you are a patient in a health care facility or when you update your medical records with your physician.]

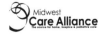 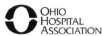 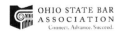

Ohio
Living Will Declaration

[R.C. §2133]

_____

(Print Full Name)

_____

(Birth Date)

This is my Living Will Declaration. I revoke all prior Living Will Declarations signed by me. I understand the nature and purpose of this document. If any provision is found to be invalid or unenforceable, it will not affect the rest of this document.

I am of sound mind and not under or subject to duress, fraud or undue influence. I am a competent adult who understands and accepts the consequences of this action. I voluntarily declare my direction that my dying not be artificially prolonged. [R.C. §2133.02 (A)(1)]

I intend that this Living Will Declaration will be honored by my family and physicians as the final expression of my legal right to refuse certain health care. [R.C.§2133.03(B)(2)]

Definitions

Adult means a person who is 18 years of age or older.

Agent or attorney-in-fact means a competent adult who a person (the "principal") can name in a Health Care Power of Attorney to make health care decisions for the principal.

Anatomical gift means a donation of part or all of a human body to take effect after the donor's death for the purpose of transplantation, therapy, research or education.

Artificially or technologically supplied nutrition or hydration means food and fluids provided through intravenous or tube feedings. *[You can refuse or discontinue a feeding tube, or authorize your Health Care Power of Attorney agent to refuse or discontinue artificial nutrition or hydration.]*

Comfort care means any measure, medical or nursing procedure, treatment or intervention, including nutrition and or hydration, that is taken to diminish a patient's pain or discomfort, but not to postpone death.

CPR means cardiopulmonary resuscitation, one of several ways to start a person's breathing or heartbeat once either has stopped. It does not include clearing a person's airway for a reason other than resuscitation.

No Expiration Date. This Living Will Declaration will have no expiration date. However, I may revoke it at any time. [R.C. §2133.04(A)]

Copies the Same as Original. Any person may rely on a copy of this document. [R.C. §2133.02(C)]

Out of State Application. I intend that this document be honored in any jurisdiction to the extent allowed by law. [R.C. §2133.14]

I have completed a **Health Care Power of Attorney**: Yes_____ No _____

Notifications. *[Note: You do not need to name anyone. If no one is named, the law requires your attending physician to make a reasonable effort to notify one of the following persons in the order named: your guardian, your spouse, your adult children who are available, your parents, or a majority of your adult siblings who are available.]*

In the event my attending physician determines that life-sustaining treatment should be withheld or withdrawn, my physician shall make a reasonable effort to notify one of the persons named below, in the following order of priority *[cross out any unused lines]*: [R.C. §2133.05(2)(a)]

First contact's name and relationship:_____

Address: _____

Telephone number(s): _____

Second contact's name and relationship:_____

Address: _____

Telephone number(s): _____

Third contact's name and relationship: _____

Address:_____

Telephone number(s): _____

X out area if not used

If I am in a **TERMINAL CONDITION** and unable to make my own health care decisions, OR if I am in a **PERMANENTLY UNCONSCIOUS STATE** and there is no reasonable possibility that I will regain the capacity to make informed decisions, then I direct my physician to let me die naturally, providing me only with **comfort care**.

For the purpose of providing comfort care, I authorize my physician to:

1. Administer no life-sustaining treatment, including CPR;
2. Withhold or withdraw artificially or technologically supplied nutrition or hydration, provided that, if I am in a permanently unconscious state, I have authorized such withholding or withdrawal under **Special Instructions** below and the other conditions have been met;
3. Issue a DNR Order; and
4. Take no action to postpone my death, providing me with only the care necessary to make me comfortable and to relieve pain.

Special Instructions.

By placing my initials, signature, check or other mark in this box, I specifically authorize my physician to withhold, or if treatment has commenced, to withdraw, consent to the provision of artificially or technologically supplied nutrition or hydration if I am in a permanently unconscious state AND my physician and at least one other physician who has examined me have determined, to a reasonable degree of medical certainty, that artificially or technologically supplied nutrition and hydration will not provide comfort to me or relieve my pain. [R.C. §2133.02(A)(3) and R.C. §2133.08]

Additional instructions or limitations.

> *[If the space below is not sufficient, you may attach additional pages.*
> *If you do not have any additional instructions or limitations, write "None" below.]*

[The "anatomical gift" language provided below is required by ORC §2133.07(C). Donate Life Ohio recommends that you indicate your authorization to be an organ, tissue or cornea donor at the Ohio Bureau of Motor Vehicles when receiving a driver license or, if you wish to place restrictions on your donation, on a Donor Registry Enrollment Form (attached) sent to the Ohio Bureau of Motor Vehicles.]

[If you use this living will to declare your authorization, indicate the organs and/or tissues you wish to donate and cross out any purposes for which you do not authorize your donation to be used. Please see the attached Donor Registry Enrollment Form for help in this regard. In all cases, let your family know your declared wishes for donation.]

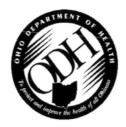

DO NOT RESUSCITATE (DNR): FREQUENTLY ASKED QUESTIONS

WHAT DOES DNR MEAN?

DNR stands for "do not resuscitate." A person who does not wish to have cardiopulmonary resuscitation (CPR) performed may make this wish known through a physician's order called a DNR order. A DNR order addresses the various methods used to revive people whose hearts have stopped functioning or who have stopped breathing. Examples of these treatments include chest compressions, electric heart shock, artificial breathing tubes and special drugs. These standardized DNR orders allow patients to choose the extent of the treatment they wish to receive at the end of life. A patient may choose to be DNR Comfort Care (DNRCC) or a DNR Comfort Care – Arrest (DNRCC-Arrest).

DOES OHIO HAVE A LAW CONCERNING DNR ORDERS?

Yes. Ohio adopted a law concerning DNR orders in 1998.

HOW CAN I GET A DNR ORDER?

An individual may obtain a DNRCC by consulting with their physician, certified nurse practitioner, certified nurse specialist, or physician assistant regarding end-of-life issues. The DNRCC allows this specific DNR order to be used in multiple settings and practice areas including, but not limited to, nursing facilities, residential care facilities, hospitals, outpatient areas, homes and public places. For a DNR order to be useful in multiple settings, it must be recognizable by health care workers. The Ohio Department of Health (ODH) has developed a standard form that is recognized throughout the health care community in Ohio. Unlike a living will and health care power of attorney, a DNR order must be written and signed by a physician, certified nurse practitioner, certified nurse specialist, or physician assistant in consultation with the patient.

WHAT IS THE DNR PROTOCOL?

The DNR protocol lists the specific actions paramedics, emergency medical technicians, physicians or nurses may take when attending to a DNR patient. The protocol also specifies actions that will not be implemented. The standard DNR protocol is to be used for a patient whose physician, certified nurse practitioner, certified nurse specialist, or physician assistant has written a DNR order.

THE DNR PROTOCOL – WHEN IS IT ACTIVATED?

Under the DNR protocol, a patient must choose between DNRCC and DNRCC – Arrest status, which in turn, determines when the DNR protocol is activated:

1) DNR Comfort Care (DNRCC) – a person receives any care that eases pain and suffering, but no resuscitative measures to save or sustain life. This protocol is activated immediately when a valid DNR order is issued or when a living will requesting no CPR becomes effective.

2) DNR Comfort Care – Arrest (DNRCC-Arrest) – a person receives standard medical care until the time he or she experiences a cardiac or respiratory arrest. Standard medical care may include cardiac monitoring or intubation prior to the occurrence of cardiac or respiratory arrest. This protocol is activated when the patient has a cardiac or respiratory arrest.

"Cardiac arrest" means absence of a palpable pulse. "Respiratory arrest" means absence of spontaneous respirations or presence of agonal breathing.

Once the protocol is activated, the health care provider

WILL:

* Suction the airway
* Administer oxygen
* Position for comfort
* Splint or immobilize
* Control bleeding
* Provide pain medication
* Provide emotional support
* Contact other providers: hospice, home health, attending physicians/CNP/CNS/PA

WILL NOT:

* Administer chest compressions
* Insert artifical airway
* Administer resuscitative drugs
* Defibrillate or cardiovert
* Provide respiratory assistance (other than that listed above)
* Initiate resuscitative IV
* Initiate cardiac monitoring

DOES DNR COMFORT CARE MEAN "DO NOT TREAT?"

The DNRCC protocol is very specific in terms of what treatment is to be given and what treatment is to be withheld. Only those items listed on the "will not" list are to be withheld. The items listed on the "will" list, along with any other treatment that may be needed for the patient's condition, may be provided as appropriate.

CAN I SIGN MY OWN DNR ORDER?
No. A DNR order must be written and signed by a physician,certified nurse practitioner, certified nurse specialist, or physician assitant in consultation with the patient.

CAN ANYONE ELSE OVERRIDE MY WISHES ABOUT CPR EVEN THOUGH A VALID DNR ORDER EXISTS?

No. You have the right to make your own decisions about your health care. If you are not able to express your wishes, other people such as a legal guardian, a person you name as your health care power of attorney, or a family member can speak for you. You should make sure these people know your desires about CPR and that you have a DNR order.

WHAT IF I CHANGE MY MIND AFTER MY PHYSICIAN WRITES A DNR ORDER?

You always have the right to change your mind and request CPR. If you do change your mind, you should talk with your physician right away about revoking your DNR order. You should also tell your family and caregivers about your decision.

IF I AM NOT ABLE TO DECIDE ABOUT CPR FOR MYSELF, WHO WILL DECIDE?

First, two doctors must determine that you are unable to decide about CPR. You will be told of this determination and have the right to object.

If you become unable to decide about CPR, and you did not tell your doctor or others about your wishes in advance, a DNR order can be written with the consent of someone chosen by you, by a family member or by a close friend. The person highest on the following list will decide about CPR for you:

- The person chosen by you to make health care decisions
- A court-appointed guardian
- Your closest relative (spouse, child, parent, sibling)
- Close friend

UNDER WHAT CIRCUMSTANCES CAN A FAMILY MEMBER OR CLOSE FRIEND DECIDE A DNR ORDER SHOULD BE WRITEN?

A family member or close friend can consent to a DNR order only when you are unable to decide for yourself and you have not appointed someone to decide for you. Your family member or close friend can consent to a DNR order when:

- You are terminally ill
- You are permanently unconscious
- CPR will not work (would be medically futile)
- CPR would impose an extraordinary burden on you given your medical condition and the expected outcome of CPR

Anyone deciding for you must base the decision on your wishes, including your religious and moral beliefs, or if your wishes are not known, on your best interests.

HOW DOES SOMEONE KNOW I AM A DNR COMFORT CARE PATIENT?

Your DNR order can serve as evidence you are a DNRCC patient and you desire the statewide standard DNR protocol to be used at the appropriate time. A wallet ID card,hospital type wristband, and DNR jewelry items such as necklaces or bracelets are also available to identify you as a DNRCC patient. You are not required to carry the ID card or to wear an identification item. However, if a provider cannot identify you as a DNRCC patient, all efforts to resuscitate you and to sustain life will be applied as this is an appropriate and legal response in the absence of definitive DNR identification.

Under the law, emergency medical services (EMS) workers are not required to search patients for DNR identification. However, if DNR identification is discovered, the EMS personnel must make reasonable efforts to verify the patient's identity. After verification, the workers must honor the DNR directive and follow the DNR protocol. The law provides immunity to EMS workers who follow the DNR directive.

WHERE CAN I GET A DNR COMFORT CARE WALLET ID CARD, BRACELET, OR OTHER IDENTIFICATION?
The DNRCC wallet ID card may be available from you physician certified nurse practitioner, certified nurse specialist, or physician assistant. The DNRCC hospital type identification wristband (bracelet) is available from hospitals, nursing homes and any other source with the capability to fabricate this type of bracelet. The format for the wallet ID card, hospital type bracelet,and a listing of retailers who MAY be able to supply DNR jewelry items is available on the DNR program webpage at: http:// www.odh.ohio.gov/odhprograms/dspc/dnr/dnr1.aspx.

DNR-freq-quest   rev 06/17/2015

HIPAA PERMITS DISCLOSURE OF POLST TO OTHER HEALTH CARE PROVIDERS AS NECESSARY

Physician Orders for Life-Sustaining Treatment

Last Name - First Name - Middle Initial

Date of Birth   Last 4 #SSN   Gender

M   F

FIRST follow these orders, **THEN** contact physician, nurse practitioner or PA-C. The POLST form is always voluntary. The POLST is a set of medical orders intended to guide medical treatment based on a person's current medical condition and goals. Any section not completed implies full treatment for that section. Everyone shall be treated with dignity and respect.

Medical Conditions/Patient Goals:

Agency Info/Sticker

A
Check One

CARDIOPULMONARY RESUSCITATION (CPR): Person has no pulse and is not breathing.

☐ CPR/Attempt Resuscitation   ☐ DNAR/Do Not Attempt Resuscitation (Allow Natural Death)

Choosing DNAR will include appropriate comfort measures and may still include the range of treatments below. When not in cardiopulmonary arrest, go to part B.

B
Check One

MEDICAL INTERVENTIONS: Person has pulse and/or is breathing.

☐ **COMFORT MEASURES ONLY** Use medication by any route, positioning, wound care and other measures to relieve pain and suffering. Use oxygen, oral suction and manual treatment of airway obstruction as needed for comfort.   **Patient prefers no hospital transfer:** *EMS contact medical control to determine if transport indicated to provide adequate comfort.*

☐ **LIMITED ADDITIONAL INTERVENTIONS** Includes care described above. Use medical treatment, IV fluids and cardiac monitor as indicated. Do not use intubation or mechanical ventilation. May use less invasive airway support (e.g. CPAP, BiPAP).   **Transfer** *to hospital if indicated. Avoid intensive care if possible.*

☐ **FULL TREATMENT** Includes care described above. Use intubation, advanced airway interventions, mechanical ventilation, and cardioversion as indicated.   **Transfer** *to hospital if indicated. Includes intensive care.*

Additional Orders: (e.g. dialysis, etc.) _____

C

SIGNATURES: The signatures below verify that these orders are consistent with the patient's medical condition, known preferences and best known information. If signed by a surrogate, the patient must be decisionally incapacitated and the person signing is the legal surrogate.

Discussed with:
☐ Patient   ☐ Parent of Minor
☐ Guardian with Health Care Authority
☐ Spouse/Other as authorized by RCW 7.70.065
☐ Health Care Agent (DPOAHC)

PRINT — Physician/ARNP/PA-C Name | Phone Number

✗ Physician/ARNP/PA-C Signature *(mandatory)* | Date *(mandatory)*

PRINT — Patient or Legal Surrogate Name | Phone Number

✗ Patient or Legal Surrogate Signature *(mandatory)* | Date *(mandatory)*

Person has: ☐ Health Care Directive (living will)
☐ Durable Power of Attorney for Health Care

Encourage all advance care planning documents to accompany POLST

SEND ORIGINAL FORM WITH PERSON WHENEVER TRANSFERRED OR DISCHARGED

Revised 4/2014   Photocopies and faxes of signed POLST forms are legal and valid. May make copies for records.
For more information on POLST visit www.wsma.org/polst.

Washington **WSMA**
State **Medical**
Association
Physician Driven
Patient Focused

 Washington State Department of
Health

HIPAA PERMITS DISCLOSURE OF POLST TO OTHER HEALTH CARE PROVIDERS AS NECESSARY

Other Contact Information (Optional)

Name of Guardian, Surrogate or other Contact Person	Relationship	Phone Number	
Name of Health Care Professional Preparing Form	Preparer Title	Phone Number	Date Prepared

D NON-EMERGENCY MEDICAL TREATMENT PREFERENCES

ANTIBIOTICS:

☐ No antibiotics. Use other measures to relieve symptoms. ☐ Use antibiotics if life can be prolonged.
☐ Determine use or limitation of antibiotics when infection occurs, with comfort as goal.

MEDICALLY ASSISTED NUTRITION:
Always offer food and liquids by mouth if feasible.

☐ Trial period of medically assisted nutrition by tube.
(Goal: _____)

☐ No medically assisted nutrition by tube. ☐ Long-term medically assisted nutrition by tube.

ADDITIONAL ORDERS: (e.g. dialysis, blood products, implanted cardiac devices, etc. Attach additional orders if necessary.)

✗ Physician/ARNP/PA-C Signature	Date
✗ Patient or Legal Surrogate Signature	Date

DIRECTIONS FOR HEALTH CARE PROFESSIONALS

Completing POLST

- The POLST is usually for persons with serious illness or frailty.
- Completing a POLST form is always voluntary.
- The POLST must be completed by a health care provider based on the patient's preferences and medical condition.
- POLST must be signed by a physician/ARNP/PA-C and patient, or their surrogate, to be valid. Verbal orders are acceptable with follow-up signature by physician/ARNP/PA-C in accordance with facility/community policy.

Using POLST

Any incomplete section of POLST implies full treatment for that section.

This POLST is valid in all care settings including hospitals until replaced by new physician's orders.

The POLST is a set of medical orders. The most recent POLST replaces all previous orders.

The POLST does not replace an advance directive. An advance directive is encouraged for all competent adults regardless of their health status. An advance directive allows a person to document in detail his/her future health care instructions and/or name a surrogate decision maker to speak on his/her behalf. When available, all documents should be reviewed to ensure consistency, and the forms updated appropriately to resolve any conflicts.

SECTION A:
- No defibrillator should be used on a person who has chosen "Do Not Attempt Resuscitation."

SECTION B:
- When comfort cannot be achieved in the current setting, the person, including someone with "Comfort Measures Only," should be transferred to a setting able to provide comfort (e.g., treatment of a hip fracture).
- An IV medication to enhance comfort may be appropriate for a person who has chosen "Comfort Measures Only."
- Treatment of dehydration is a measure which may prolong life. A person who desires IV fluids should indicate "Limited Additional Interventions" or "Full Treatment."

SECTION D:
- Oral fluids and nutrition must always be offered if medically feasible.

Reviewing POLST

This POLST should be reviewed periodically whenever:
(1) The person is transferred from one care setting or care level to another, or
(2) There is a substantial change in the person's health status, or
(3) The person's treatment preferences change.

A competent adult, or the surrogate of a person who is not competent, can void the form and request alternative treatment.

To void this form, draw line through "Physician Orders" and write "VOID" in large letters. Any changes require a new POLST.

Review of this POLST Form

Review Date	Reviewer	Location of Review	Review Outcome		
			☐ No Change		
			☐ Form Voided	☐ New form completed	
			☐ No Change		
			☐ Form Voided	☐ New form completed	

SEND ORIGINAL FORM WITH PERSON WHENEVER TRANSFERRED OR DISCHARGED

Photocopies and faxes of signed POLST forms are legal and valid. May make copies for records. **OVER ▶**
For more information on POLST visit www.wsma.org/polst.

Where I Got My Information

Many of my sources for "Nine Important Lessons" are cited in the text. For those that are not, I've listed them below. You can find most of these by searching the Internet.

Lesson 1   Find Out What You Don't Know

1.   "Conversations That Light the Way," The Ohio End of Life Cooperative, Leadingageohio.org.

Lesson 2   Make the Most of a Doctor Visit

2.   "High Blood Pressure Unique to Older Adults," American Geriatrics Society, healthinaging.org .

3.   "Shared Decision Making - Finding the Sweet Spot," Terri R. Fried, M.D. *New England Journal of Medicine*, January 14, 2016.

4.   "The Physician Employment Trend: What You Need to Know," Travis Singleton, Phillip Miller. *Family Practice Management*, July-August, 2015.

5.   "The Case for Concierge Medicine," Richard Gunderman, M.D. *The Atlantic*, July 16, 2014.

Lesson 3   Be Their Voice

6.   "Epidemiologic study of in-hospital cardiopulmonary resuscitation in the elderly," William J. Ehlenbach, M.D., et al. *New England Journal of Medicine*, July 2, 2009.

7.   "Do Not Resuscitate (DNR): Frequently Asked Questions," Ohio Department of Health, odh.ohio.gov/odhprograms .

8.   "Avoid potential pitfalls of living wills, DNR, and POLST with checklists, standardization," Ferdinando L. Mirarchi, DO, FACEP. *ACEP Now*, May 9, 2014.

9.   "Physician Orders for Life-Sustaining Treatment," Washington State Medical Association, www.wsma.org.

Where I Got My Information (cont'd)

Lesson 4   First, Do No Harm

10. "Screening Mammography in Older Women: A Review,"
     Louise C. Walter, M.D. and Mara A. Schonberg, M.D.
     Journal of the American Medical Association, April 2, 2014.

11. *"How Healthy is Your Doctor,"* Dr. Kathryn Collins, F.A.C.E.P.
     White Grass Press, 2013.

12. "Adverse drug reactions in elderly patients", P.A.Routledge, M.S. O'Mahony, K.W.
     Woodhouse. *British Journal of Clinical Pharmacology*, 57(2), Feb., 2004.

13. "Living With C. Diff: Learning to Control the Spread of Clostridium difficile (C. diff),"
     Arizona Healthcare-Associated Infection Advisory Committee, preventHAIaz.gov .

14. "Sundowning: Late Day Confusion," Glenn Smith, PhD.
     Mayoclinic.org, March 27, 2014.

15. "Geriatric Chest Imaging: When and How to Image the Elderly Lung,
     Age-Related Changes, and Common Pathologies," J. Gossner, R. Nau.
     Radiology Research and Practice, July 1, 2013.

16. "Switch Over from Intravenous to Oral Therapy: A Concise Overview,"
     Cyriac JM and James E. *Journal of Pharmocology and Pharmaocotherapeutics*,
     April 5, 2014.

17. "Sticking Points—How to Handle Difficult Blood Draws,"
     Anne Paxton. College of American Pathologists, March 2011.

18. "Blood Clot Treatments, Anticoagulants: Treatment of Blood Clots,"
     National Blood Clot Alliance, stoptheclot.org.

19. "Unnecessary Urinary Catheterizations and Lack of Informed Consent,"
     patientmodesty.org.

20. "The surprising dangers of CT scans and X-rays,"
     Consumer Reports, January 25, 2015.

21. *"How Healthy is Your Doctor,"* Dr. Kathryn Collins, F.A.C.E.P.
     White Grass Press, 2013.

Where I Got My Information (cont'd)

22. "Unfair to Patients: Medicare's three-day rule,"
    Boston Globe, August 15, 2016.

23. "The Patient Wants to Leave. The Hospital Says 'No Way,'"
    Paula Span. *The New York Times*, July 7 2017.

Lesson 5   Be Ready For Rehab

24. "Deconditioning in the hospitalized elderly", A. Gillis, B. MacDonald.
    The Canadian Nurse, June, 2005, and N.I.H. PubMed.gov .

25. "Healthcare Associated Infections," Centers for Disease Control and Infections,
    cdc.gov/hai/surveillance/.

26. "Postoperative delirium in older adults: Best practice statement
    from the American Geriatrics Society," American Geriatrics Society
    Expert Panel on Postoperative Delirium in Older Adults.
    Journal of the American College of Surgeons, 2015.

27. "Delirium in older adults," Dennis M. Popeo, M.D.
    Mount Sinai Journal of Medicine, July, 2011.

28. "A Neuropathologic Study of 3 Population-Based Cohort Studies,"
    Daniel H. Davis, PhD, MRCP; Graciela Muniz-Terrera, PhD; Hannah A. D. Keage, PhD;
    et al. *JAMA Psychiatry*, 2017.

29. "Educating family caregivers for older adults about delirium: A systemic review,"
    Margaret J. Bull, PhD.; Lesley Boaz, PhD., RN, GNP, FNP; Martha Jerme, MSN,
    MLIS, RN. *Worldviews on Evidence-Based Nursing*, March 10, 2016.

Lesson 7   Choose the Right Place for Your Loved One

30. "Long Term Care Insurance: Is it Worth it?", Leslie Scism,
    The Wall Street Journal, May 1, 2015.

31. "Predicting the mortality of residents at admission to nursing home: A longitudinal
    cohort study," Ingibjörg Hjaltadóttir, Ingalill Rahm Hallberg, Anna Kristensson Ekwall
    and Per Nyberg. *BMC Health Services Research*, April, 2011.

Where I Got My Information (cont'd)

32. "The Meaning of 'Aging in Place' to Older People", J.Wiles, A. Leibing, N. Guberman, J. Reeve, R. Allen, *The Gerontologist*, May 2, 2012.

Lesson 8   Know When Enough is Enough

33. "Palliative Care Continues Its Annual Growth Trend: According to Latest Center to Advance Palliative Care Analysis", *Center to Advance Palliative Care*, May 27, 2015.

34. "Evaluation of the Prognostic Criteria for Medicare Hospice Eligibility", D Helen Moore. *University of South Florida Scholar Commons*, 2004.

35. "Hospice Care Helps, But Often Doctors Don't Recommend It Soon Enough", *Harvard Health Publications*, Sept. 1, 2005.

Lesson 9   Remember, It's Not Your Journey

36. "Understanding Caregiver Stress Syndrome," Sandra Tunajek, CRNA, DNP. *American Association of Nurse Anesthetists*, October, 2010.

Helpful Terms

Lesson 1   Find Out What You Don't Know

Guided Conversation - a talk with your loved one about their health care wishes, preferably before a health crisis occurs

Health Care Provider - a person providing medical care services

Tube Feedings - a tube is placed directly into the stomach through a small incision in the abdomen (or through the nose and into the stomach) to administer nutrition

Comatose - unconscious

Terminal Illness - a disease that cannot be cured and that is reasonably expected to result in the death of the patient within a short period of time

Lesson 2   Make the Most of a Doctor Visit

Congestive Heart Failure (CHF) - a condition that occurs when the heart cannot pump blood as it should

Health Care Proxy - someone a patient legally designates to speak on their behalf regarding their health care if the patient becomes physically or mentally incapable of making their own health care decisions

Health Care Agent, Health Care Surrogate, Health Care Representative or Health Care Attorney-in-Fact - see Health Care Proxy

Prognosis - the likely course of a disease or ailment

Well Visit - a scheduled appointment with one's health care provider when they are not sick

Baseline Data - a point serving as the basis for further study or comparison in a person's health

Blood Pressure - the pressure exerted by the heart to pump blood through the body

Shared Decision Making or SDM - decision making about a person's health or medical treatment that encourages equal participation by the health care provider and the patient

Medicare A - a hospital insurance that covers inpatient hospital care, skilled nursing facility, hospice, lab tests, surgery, home health care

HIPPA - "Health Insurance Portability and Accountability Act" of 1996 that established a "bill of rights" regarding patient medical records

Survival Rate - the percentage of people in a study or treatment group still alive for a given period of time after diagnosis of a particular disease

Cure Rate - the proportion of people with a disease that are cured by a given treatment, often determined by comparing disease-free survival of treated people against a matched control group that never had the disease

Informed Consent - the patient is told (or gets information in some way) about the possible risks and benefits of a treatment

Consent to treatment - see Informed Consent

Bedside Manner - doctor's approach or attitude toward a patient

Geriatrics - a specialized field of medicine that deals with the health problems of the elderly

Geriatric Psychiatry or psychogeriatrics - deals with the mental issues of patients over age sixty-five, including delirium and dementia

Delirium - an acutely disturbed state of mind that is characterized by restlessness, illusions, and incoherence of thought and speech

Dementia - a chronic or persistent mental disorder caused by brain disease or injury and marked by memory disorders, personality changes and impaired reasoning

Gerontology - the study of the impact of aging on the individual and on society, focused on increasing the quality of life of the elderly

Physician Group - several doctors who enter medical practice together as one legal entity to cut operating (billing) and liability (insurance) costs

"Personalized" or Concierge Physician Services - these physicians attempt to make preventative health care their first priority and personalize medical care for their patients

Urgent Care Clinic - often called "walk-in" clinic, it offers basic medical services without an appointment and is often open 7 days a week

Physician's Assistant (PA) - a nationally certified and state-licensed medical professional who practices medicine on health care teams and with supervision by a physician or other provider

Board Certified Physician - a physician who has not only obtained a medical license, but has also demonstrated exceptional competency in his/her particular medical field

Internist - a physician practicing Internal Medicine or general medicine dealing with the prevention, diagnosis, and treatment of adult diseases

Internal Medicine - see Internist

General Practitioner (GP) - an internist (see above) or family practice physician (who treats people of all ages) providing primary care for patients

Geriatrician - a physician who practices geriatrics

Primary Care - health care at a basic rather than specialized level for people making an initial approach to a medical professional for treatment

Baby Boomer - typically people born from the mid 1940s to the mid-1960's

Hospitalist - a physician who cares for you while you are hospitalized

Electronic Health Records (EHR) Incentive Program - a Medicare and Medicaid program which incentivizes health care providers and hospitals to make EHR available to patients

Integrative Medicine - a broad range of healing philosophies and approaches that are stand-alone alternatives or additions to conventional care

Alternative Medicine or Holistic Medicine - see Integrative Medicine

Acute Medical Care - health care where a patient receives active but short-term treatment for a severe injury or episode of illness

Acupuncture - a key component of traditional Chinese medicine and healing in which thin needles are inserted into the body

Nutritional Counseling - individual nutrition consultation that may address weight issues, chronic health conditions, meal planning or food allergies, among others

Osteopathic Manipulation - involving use of the practitioner's hands to diagnose, treat, and prevent illness or injury

Chiropractic - the diagnosis and manipulative treatment of misalignments of the joints, especially those of the spinal column, as a treatment for other disorders in the body

Stress Management - techniques to relax including breathing exercises, muscle relaxation and stretching exercises to relieve stress

Homeopathy - the treatment of disease by ingesting minute doses of natural substances that in a healthy person might produce symptoms of disease

Herbal Medicine - a type of dietary supplement using some part of an herb for its therapeutic properties

Complimentary and Alternative Medicine (CAM) - see Integrative Medicine

Western Medicine or Conventional Medicine - a system in which medical doctors and other health care professionals treat symptoms and diseases using drugs, radiation or surgery

Functional Medicine - medical practice or treatments that focus on optimal functioning of the body and its organs, usually involving systems of holistic or alternative medicine

Health Insurance Portability and Accountability Act - see HIPPA

Right to Access - part of HIPPA, it guarantees that a person has access to their protected health information (PHI) generated by any health insurance plan or health care provider

Protected Health Information (PHI) - see Right to Access

Lesson 3   Be Their Voice

Last (or Final) Will and Testament - a legal document used to manage a person's estate after their death

Durable Power of Attorney for Health Care - the person designated by a patient to be the legal authority to speak on their behalf when the patient is physically or mentally incapable of making their own health care decisions

Health Care Proxy, Health Care Attorney-in-Fact, Health Care Agent or Health Care Surrogate - see Durable Power of Attorney for Health Care

Advance Directives - typically a set of three legal documents that gives direction to those charged with the patient's well being, about how to proceed with medical care based on the patient's wishes

Living Will - a patient's direction *in writing* regarding his/her medical care, in case they are unable to communicate this at the time it's needed

Organ Donor Form - a form provided to declare a patient's intent to donate organs and tissues for such purposes as transplantation or education

Guardianship Nomination Form - a document that transfers the legal responsibility of a child to another person, typically in the event that the person can no longer care for their child

Elder Law - a specialty within the legal field that deals with a broad range of legal concerns that affect the elderly

Wills and Probate Lawyer - a type of state licensed attorney who advises personal representatives or executors and the beneficiaries of an estate on how to settle the final affairs of a deceased person

Patient Rights or Patient Bill of Rights - a few rights guaranteed by the federal government (see HIPAA), states, hospitals and medical facilities; see Informed Consent

Do Not Resuscitate (DNR) - a physician or medical facility provided document that requires hospitals to allow individuals to make decisions about their own emergency medical treatment

Vegetative State - absence of responsiveness and awareness due to overwhelming dysfunction of the cerebral hemispheres of the brain

Chest Compressions - part of CPR (cardiopulmonary resuscitation) involving hand compressions at the center of the chest to restart the beating of the heart

Patient Self-determination Act of 1991 - Most hospitals, nursing homes, home health
    agencies and HMO's are required by law to provide information on advance
    directives to patients at the time of admission

Mechanical Ventilation - helps patients breathe by assisting the inhalation of oxygen
    into the lungs and the exhalation of carbon dioxide

Electric Heart Shock - a procedure in which a brief electric shock is given to the heart
    to reset the heart rhythm back to its normal

Intubation - the placement of a flexible plastic tube into the trachea (windpipe) to
    maintain an open airway or to administer certain drugs

IV Port - when drugs cannot be given through a standard IV, a small medical appliance
    can be installed beneath the skin where a catheter connects the port to a vein

EMT (Emergency Medical Technician) - provides out of hospital emergency medical
    care and transportation for critical and emergency patients who access the
    emergency medical services (EMS) system.

**Physicians Orders for Life Sustaining Treatment or Provider Orders for Life
Sustaining Treatment (POLST)** - a "prescription" for the treatment of seriously
    ill patients in an emergency situation, based on the patient's Advance Directives,
    treatment preferences and consultation with their doctor

Medical Orders for Life Sustaining Treatment (MOLST) - see POLST

ABC's of Resuscitation - airways, breathing and circulation are stabilized in the patient

Artificial Life Support - systems that use medical technology to aid, support, or
    replace a vital function of the body that has been seriously damaged - such as
    pacemakers, defibrillators, dialysis machines and respirators

"Death With Dignity" - a law enacted in some U.S. states that gives physicians the right
    to prescribe lethal medication to terminally ill patients who have a short time to live

"Physician Aid-In-Dying" or "Physician Assisted Suicide" - see "Death With Dignity"

Resuscitation or Surgical Pause - in a medical emergency, after the doctor has
    stabilized the patient, this pause allows the doctor and the patient or health care
    proxy to discuss next steps based on the POLST, the patient's health goals and
    Advance Directives

Cardiac Arrest - a sudden, sometimes temporary, cessation of function of the heart

Respiratory Arrest - caused by apnea (cessation of breathing) due to failure of the lungs to function effectively

Cardiopulmonary Resuscitation (CPR) - an emergency technique used on someone whose heart or breathing has stopped

Artificially Supplied Nutrition or Hydration - given to a person who cannot eat or drink enough to sustain life or health, nutrition and hydration is given through an IV or tube in the stomach

Dialysis - the clinical purification of blood by dialysis, as a substitute for the normal function of the kidney

Lesson 4   First, Do No Harm

Hippocratic Oath - an oath historically taken by physicians which includes the promise "first, do no harm"

Chronic Disease - a disease lasting 3 months or more, according to the U.S. National Center for Health Statistics; and generally cannot be prevented by vaccines or cured by medication

Diagnostic Tests - a procedure performed to confirm or determine the presence of disease in an individual suspected of having the disease

Adverse Drug Reaction (ADR) - ill side effect of a medication or the combination of more than one medication

Hypertension Medication - medication to treat high blood pressure

Statin - a class of drugs often prescribed by doctors to help lower cholesterol levels in the blood

Blood Thinner - anticoagulant medication such as Warfarin (Coumadin) used to help to prevent blood clots from forming in the blood, specifically for some types of heart disease

Diuretic - also called water pills, a medication designed to expel more water and salt from the body as urine, in an attempt to lower elevated blood pressure

Osteoporosis - a medical condition in which the bones become brittle and fragile from loss of tissue, typically as a result of hormonal changes, or deficiency of calcium or vitamin D

Preventative Antibiotics - mainly prescribed for a short 'course' to treat bacterial infections or to protect against infection before surgery or other potential health trauma

Stool Softeners - used on a short-term basis to relieve constipation in people who should avoid straining during bowel movements because of heart conditions, hemorrhoids or other problems

Anti-psychotic Drugs - also known as neuroleptics or major tranquilizers, a class of medication primarily used to manage psychosis, principally in schizophrenia and bipolar disorder

Sundowning Syndrome - a state of confusion at the end of the day and into the night, fairly common in people with some form of dementia

Alzheimer's Disease - a type of dementia that causes problems with memory, thinking and behavior and accounts for 60 to 80 percent of dementia cases

Vascular Dementia - the second most common type of dementia, caused by a series of small strokes over a long period and affects memory, thinking, language, judgment, and behavior

Second Opinion - when a health care provider recommends surgery or a major procedure or treatment, the patient can opt to get another medical expert's opinion

Observation - a patient brought to the hospital emergency room who is not well enough to go home but not sick enough to be formally admitted to the hospital for treatment, may be kept overnight at the hospital and billed as an outpatient

Hospital Admission - a patient who is admitted to the hospital as an inpatient and is now considered covered by their medical insurance based on their policy's requirements

The Notice Act - a new federal law scheduled to go into effect in 2016 requiring hospitals to notify patients after twenty-four hours if they are still on "observation" rather than "admission"

Routine Procedures - medical procedures that are ordered for a patient in a hospital or other medical setting on a frequent or daily basis due to facility policy but are not essential for the individual patient's treatment plan

Intravenous Medications (IVs) - medications delivered directly into the patient's vein using a needle or tube

Phlebotomy - the act of drawing blood from a patient for clinical or medical testing, transfusions, donations, or research

Peripherally Inserted Central Catheters (PICC lines) - a thin, soft, long tube that is inserted into the arm, leg or neck of the patient and into a large vein that carries blood to the heart; used for long-term antibiotics, nutrition or medications, and blood draws

Ultrasound Scan (Sonogram) - a procedure that uses high-frequency sound waves to create an image of part of the inside of the body

Echocardiogram - a scan that uses ultrasound waves to investigate the action of the heart

Invasive Medical Procedure - a medical procedure that invades (enters) the body, usually by cutting or puncturing the skin or by inserting instruments into the body

Non-Invasive Medical Procedure - a conservative procedure that at the very least does not require cutting into the body or removing tissue

Minimally-Invasive Medical Procedure - a variety of techniques used by physicians to operate on a patient with less damage to the body than with open surgery

Laparoscopic Surgery - a surgical procedure in which a fiber-optic instrument is inserted through the abdominal wall to view the organs in the abdomen or to permit a surgical procedure

CT or CAT Scan - a special X-ray test that produce cross-sectional images of the body using X- rays and a computer

Positron Emission Tomography (PET scan) - an imaging test used for checking diseases in the body by injecting a special dye with radioactive tracers into a vein in the patient's arm and then the organs and tissues absorb the tracer

Magnetic Resonance Imaging (MRI) - uses a large magnet and radio waves to look at organs and structures inside the body

AMA (Against Medical Advice) - a patient or their health care proxy goes against the doctor's advice and refuses a treatment or medical procedure or admission to a health care facility

Lesson 5   Be Ready For Rehab

Ambulatory - able to walk

Cardiac or Coronary Unit - a hospital ward specialized in the care of patients with heart conditions that require continuous monitoring and treatment

Physical Therapy (PT) - a specialty in Western Medicine that uses mechanical force and movements to promote mobility and increase quality of life in the physically impaired

Occupational Therapy (OT) - the assessment and intervention to develop, recover, or maintain the meaningful activities or occupation of the patient

Deconditioning - physiological change following a period of inactivity, bedrest or sedentary lifestyle resulting in functional losses of mental status, continence and activities of daily living, and frequently associated with hospitalization in the elderly

Rehabilitation Facility (IRF) - often an in-patient facility for those with conditions like stroke or a brain injury, who need an intensive rehabilitation program

Hospital Delirium - patients with dementia or in frail health may experience delirium due to surgery, infection, isolation, dehydration, poor nutrition or medications such as painkillers, sedatives and sleeping pills

Urinary Tract Infection (UTI) - an infection in any part of the urinary system, the kidneys, bladder, or urethra

Hypoxia - deficiency in the amount of oxygen reaching the tissues

Electrolyte Imbalance - electrolytes are a group of essential salts that are needed for bodily function and a level too high or too low can cause symptoms such as irregular heartbeat

Physical Restraints - anything near or on the body which restricts movement, i.e. bed rails or belts, which keep people confined to their beds

Urinary Catheterization - a hollow, partially flexible tube that is inserted into the patient's bladder to collect their urine into a drainage bag

Iatrogenic Events - a negative medical event induced inadvertently by a physician or surgeon or by a medical treatment or diagnostic procedure

Cognitive Orientation - a person's ability to identify person, place, and time accurately

Mobility - the ability to move or be moved freely and easily

Skilled Nursing/Rehab facility (SNF) or Skilled Nursing Unit (SNU) - a health care institution that provides supervision of the care of every patient by a physician and at least one registered nurse

Speech-Language Pathology - a field of expertise specializing in the evaluation, diagnosis, and treatment of communication disorders, voice disorders and swallowing

Acute Care - providing or concerned with short-term, usually immediate medical care, as for serious illness or traumatic injury

Sub-Acute Care - complex patient care or rehabilitation in SNFs rather than the hospital

Care Conference - for patients in long-term facilities, similar to a rounding

Rounding - in a short-term care facility, the clinical staff move from room to room at a specific time on a specific day to involve each patient and their family in discussions about progress, treatment options and discharge plans

Medicare Advantage Plan (MAP) or Gap Insurance - a private insurance policy that covers some or all of the cost of acute medical care not covered by Medicare

Medicare Savings Program - certain U.S. states have this program that may help with Medicare premiums, deductibles and coinsurance

Medicaid - a combined federal and state run program, currently only rarely being used for short- term rehab and nursing home stays

Lesson 6   Consider Bringing Them Home

Home Medical Care, Home Health Care or Home Rehabilitation - registered nurses, physical therapists, occupational therapists, home health aides come to the home to help those who are recovering after a hospital or facility stay, or need additional support to remain at home and avoid unnecessary hospitalization

Lesson 7   Choose the Right Place for Your Loved One

Alzheimer Special Care Units or Memory Care Units (SCUs) - isolated wards, floors or units of a SNF that address the medical issues of patients with dementia

Continuing Care Retirement Communities (CCRC) - retirement communities that offer more than one kind of housing and different levels of care where residents move from one level to another based on their needs

Residential Care Homes (Adult Family Homes, Board and Care Homes, Small Group Homes) - often a single-family dwelling in neighborhoods, these facilities provide non-medical care for the elderly

Assisted Living Facility - provides help with some activities of daily living and personal care to residents who live in their own apartments and eat in communal arrangements.

Reverse Mortgage - a home equity loan that pays you cash for the value of your home without selling it

Accelerated Death Benefits - a tax-free advance on a life insurance policy for those people with terminal illnesses

Life Settlements - a person can sell their life insurance policy for cash

Vatical Settlements - a company buys a person's life insurance policy, pays their premiums, and pays out a percentage to the owner

Immediate Annuity - a person makes a single payment to an insurance company and they send back a guaranteed monthly amount

Deferred Annuity - a person makes a single payment in exchange for monthly payments for long-term care and a deferred cash fund

Long-Term Care or Extended Care (LTCF) - nursing homes, skilled nursing facilities or assisted living facilities providing a variety of services, both medical and personal care, to people who are unable to manage independently in the community

Aging in Place - a person's desire to continue living in their own home as they age, rather than moving to an assisted living or other institutional arrangement

Private Duty Home Care or Custodial Care - a nurse aide or home care worker comes into the home for specified hours or days at a time to relieve the caregivers and provide necessary support to the patient with hygiene tasks, household chores and companionship

Nurse Aide (NA) - working under the supervision of nurses or physicians, they address most fundamental elements of a patient's care, i.e., feed, dress, bathe and groom patients

Long-term Care Health Insurance - an insurance program that became popular in the 1980s and 90s, and was intended to cover the cost of assisted living or in-home professional care toward the end of one's life

Lesson 8   Know When Enough is Enough

Aggressive Treatment - a particular approach to a life-threatening illness or condition whereby the patient will receive every medication or treatment that doctors can devise to treat his or her illness

Prognosis - the likely course of a disease or ailment

Teaching Hospitals - a hospital or medical center that provides clinical education and training to future and current health professionals

Palliative Care - a medical approach to improve the quality of life of patients facing life-threatening illness, i.e., the prevention and relief of suffering

210   *"Helpful Resources"*

How to Find Things In This Book

The Patient/Doctor Relationship, 47
Dr. Hanzelik On Improving the Patient Experience, 49
Dr. Hanzelik On Learning to Communicate With a Physician, 54
Dr. Hanzelik On Treating the "Whole Patient", 57

Treatment Vs. Trauma, 63
Dr. Hanzelik On the Trauma of Being Admitted to a Hospital, 65
Dr. Hanzelik On Choosing the Best Treatment Options, 70
Dr. Hanzelik On the Crucial Role of Patient Rehabilitation, 75
Dr. Hanzelik On the Challenges of Caregiving, 78

A Voice Not A Victim, 81
Dr. Hanzelik On Having a Voice in One's Medical Care, 83
Dr. Hanzelik On the Effectiveness of Advance Directives, 89
Dr. Hanzelik On Relieving the Patient's Suffering, 92

Nine Important Lessons, 99

Find Out What You Don't Know, 103
A Guided Conversation, 104

Make the Most of a Doctor Visit, 105
An Effective Doctor Visit, 105
Shared Decision Making, 106
What is Geriatrics?, 108
Examining "Physician Groups", 109
"Personalized" Physician Services, 110
Integrative Medicine, A New Alternative, 111
Who's Heard of HIPAA?, 112
HIPAA's Right to Access, 112
HIPAA's Privacy Rule, 114

Be Their Voice, 115
What Are Advanced Directives?, 115
"Durable Power of Attorney for Health Care", 116
Responsibilities of a Health Care Proxy, 117
Living Will, 117
Where to Find Advance Directives Forms, 119
Do Not Resuscitate (DNR), 119
POLST or MOLST, 121
Do Advance Directives Really Work?, 123

Does Elder Law Help?, 124
Is There Something Called Patient Rights?, 127
"Informed Consent", 127

First, Do No Harm, 128
Prevent, Cure or Manage Disease?, 129
ADRs (Adverse Drug Reactions), 130
Clostridium difficile (C. diff), 131
Sundowning Syndrome, 132
Alternatives (or Supplementation) to Western Medicine, 133
What is Meant by "Aggressive Care"?, 135
Invasive Medical Treatment, 135
Non-invasive Medical Treatment, 135
"Routine" Medical Procedures, 137
"Observation" versus "Admission", 138
When Is It Time To Get a Second Opinion?, 140
AMA (Against Medical Advice), 140

Be Ready For Rehab, 141
What Is Deconditioning?, 142
Other Reasons for Rehab, 142
"Hospital Delirium", 143
Skilled Nursing Rehab, 145
The Social Worker's Role, 148
A Care Conference or "Rounding", 149
Paying For Rehab, 150
Medicaid and Rehab, 151

Consider Bringing Them Home, 153
Medical Coverage for Home Rehabilitation, 153
Evaluating Home Health Care, 154

Choose the Right Place For Your Loved One, 157
Long-term Care Facilities, 157
Continuing Care Retirement Communities (CCRC), 159
Assisted Living Facilities, 160
Nursing Homes, 160
Residential Care Homes, 160
Alzheimer Special Care Facilities, 161
Paying for Long-term Care, 161
Long-term Care Insurance, 162
Life Insurance Options, 163

Annuities, 163
Reverse Mortgages, 163
Life Expectancy and Long-term Care Facilities, 164
Aging in Place, 165
Private Duty Home Care, 166

Know When Enough Is Enough, 168
Palliative Care, 169
Hospice, 170
When to Request Hospice, 171
Paying for Hospice, 172
Qualifying for Hospice, 172
What to Expect From a Hospice Program, 173

Remember, It's Not Your Journey, 176
Caregiver Stress Syndrome, 176
Parting Thoughts, 177

Helpful Resources, 181
Sample of "Living Will", 183
"DNR" Frequently Asked Questions, 187
Sample of "POLST", 191
 Where I Got My Information, 193
Helpful Terms, 197

Dr. Hanzelik On The Future of Medicine 217

About Llee Sivitz

As a kid, I loved to write. In fact, when I was nine years old, I "published" a newspaper and my first headline heralded the arrival of a neighbor's new litter of kittens. Sadly, the newspaper folded after only two editions because I hand-printed each copy and subsequently suffered from a severe case of writer's cramp.

Years later, as a student at the University of Florida, my college counselor advised me to major in something "I was good at." So, although I had a passion for art, I decided to major in journalism. I learned a lot about writing, and a lot about what I didn't know about life. One particular day, my News Writing class was cancelled because my professor had committed suicide. I heard later that he left a suicide note in his typewriter. I'm sure it was well written.

Eventually, I met my husband and we moved to his hometown of Cincinnati, Ohio, where we raised our two sons. On a lark, I submitted a story to our local newspaper about my misadventures while attempting to walk in our local running marathon (evidently, walking solo was not allowed.) To my delight and amazement, the newspaper picked up the story - and offered me a job. (And the next year, the marathon allowed individual walkers to participate!)

I loved being a news reporter, and tried to be an agent for change in a city that rarely saw people walking or running. I filed over two hundred stories as a fitness writer and covered exercise trends like hot yoga and race walking; interviewed national celebrities like Richard Simmons and Montel Williams; and had my readers follow along as I got "trained" by a local trainer. However, like many caregivers of aged parents, when Mom's illnesses became the priority, my news writing career came to a grinding halt.

Today, I continue to pursue my interest in natural healing, and I currently own a whole food nutritional products franchise. But whenever I can, I try to use my writing to help others feel empowered to help themselves. You can connect with me at SpeakingUpForMom.com or Speaking Up For Mom on Facebook or by email at speakingupformom@gmail.com.

It Takes a Village...

I'd like to thank the following people who encouraged and supported me in the writing of this book:

James Sivitz, my sweetest man and first editor, who has been with me through thick and thin and always appreciates my writing;

Lumen Sivitz, my older son, who first gave me the honor of being called "Mom" and whose enthusiasm for my endeavors is priceless;

Axis Sivitz, my younger son, a natural born teacher who teaches me more than he can ever realize, and my social media mentor for this book;

Dianne Brown, a memorable friend who first encouraged me to write this book and fittingly, gave me its first "like" on Facebook;

Dale Stoops, a friend and printing consultant whose genuine interest in the project contributed to my second wind to finish the book;

Dana Studt, a dear friend whose love and experience of the elderly made her a perfect sounding board, and who inspired me to reorganize the book to be more readable and to seek out the best references;

Melinda Zemper, a skillful writer and marketing maven whose kind and timely suggestions were invaluable, including her recommendation that I change the book title (which was not easy) and pointing out the logical gaps in Mom's story and imploring me to not be "so hard on yourself";

Alexandria Poon, R.N., a group leader for caregiving resources who provided valuable updates on how things have changed since Mom's health care journey (and how things haven't);

Kathryn Collins, M.D., F.A.C.E.P., whose insights as an Emergency Medicine Physician and fellow author provided unique and important feedback, both medically and making me aware of unnecessary use of my "cynical" voice;

Dr. Edward Hanzelik, Board Certified Internist, *Speaking Up For Mom* contributing author and medical consultant, for his kind empathy to me regarding Mom's story and his clarity and passion as a physician that brought the book's purpose to life;

And Prem Rawat, for his love and guidance throughout my life's journey.

And to all of you who have said, "Please let me know when you have published your book," I thank you for affirming that this book is needed.

About Dr. Edward Hanzelik

While in high school, I started thinking about what career I wanted to pursue, and the first thing I thought was, "I will become a lawyer."

So after graduating from high school, I took a summer job with a very prominent law firm on Wall Street and quickly discovered that I did NOT want to be a lawyer. It was too much paperwork!

Then I decided to look into medicine, and began volunteering at a local hospital. I enjoyed being with the people I met in that environment and it was really upon this basis that I decided to become a doctor. I had had very few experiences with physicians prior to that time, and no one else in my family had ever been a doctor. But I think I made a wonderful decision and to this day I am very grateful for it.

Yet, from the very beginning of my medical career, even during my physician's training, I hoped to get more out of the practice of medicine than the practice of medicine was offering. In fact, in my last year of residency I took several non-required courses such as "Talking to Patients Who are Dying," and "Doing Psychotherapy for Patients" - trying to learn different things to help patients through their crises.

During that time, I was also in charge of an entire medical floor at Beth Israel Hospital in Boston, and I oversaw interns, residents and attending doctors. We would routinely do patient "rounds" where a team of thirty people, all in white coats, would gather around a person's bed and go over their test results, where they were in their care, and what was going to happen next. It was really quite impressive.

However, I also did my own rounds, usually on Saturday or Sunday mornings, and I visited each of the patients on my floor. These soon became known as the "cry rounds" because the patients would often start crying! I would hold their hands and listen to their experiences and hear how was it for them. And I could see how painful and difficult it was, and it really influenced my practice as a doctor. It was during this time that I started looking for a deeper understanding of life, and thankfully I found ways to go inside and have an inner experience of what I was looking for.

When I finished my residency at Beth Israel, I searched the want ads and found a job as a doctor for Glacier National Park in Montana. That was my first job as a physician - as a summer doctor for the park. I had a little cabin to live in, right next to the clinic. And in the winter, it would snow so much that the snow would be as high as the roof of the cabin! But it was a wonderful way to launch my career. And it's been very exciting and enjoyable ever since.

Note: Dr. Hanzelik's first co-authored book is *The Inner Game of Stress: Outsmart Life's Challenges and Fulfill Your Potential.*

Dr. Hanzelik, what would you like to say regarding the future of medicine in the U.S?

I went to a conference in Arizona and it was about the future of medicine. The speakers talked about completely transforming the practice of medicine. The human body has around twenty thousand genes, and you can have your whole "genome" analyzed to see what your genetic makeup can tell you about your body. So there's all sorts of things that are becoming very individual, like what medicines a person should or shouldn't take, and some of that determination is genetically based. In fact, what foods a person should eat or avoid could eventually depend on their genetics. So there's this vast array of information in our genome that is hardly being used by doctors. And these futurists are envisioning that eventually the first thing a doctor will do is pull up your genome and match it with your symptoms to come up with an individualized prescription based on your genetic makeup.

And then there's the whole study of "epigenetics," which is very interesting. It explores not only how your genes can indicate a trajectory of your health, but whether those genes will activate or not based on other factors like diet, stress, etc. So your lifestyle choices may determine whether a genetic condition actually ends up expressing itself in you the way it does in other members of your family.

In fact, not only will physicians be looking at your genome, they will also do a complete analysis of your "microbiome." We have more bacteria in our gut (or digestive system) than we have cells in our body! The image of ourselves being filled up with bacteria as a way of functioning may not be very appealing. But that is the way it is. And if you take an antibiotic for an infection, for instance, it completely changes your microbiome almost immediately. So scientists are working really hard to try and understand what the microbiome can tell us, and it's clear that it's an important factor in our health.

In your opinion, are doctors today happy with their profession or is there discontent, and why?

There is a great deal of discontent among doctors. And one reason is the real essence of being a doctor is no longer taught. A partner in my medical practice told me that one of his professors said, "Doctors deal with the most intimate concerns of people, yet doctors are not prepared for it." Many physicians don't learn how to communicate; they don't learn how to feel for a person; they don't learn about empathy and kindness and compassion. Doctors have to go elsewhere to learn these things. Luckily, some know it naturally and that's wonderful. But many do not. And that is not only a problem, but it makes their practice of medicine very unsatisfying.

What would your advice be to those just graduating from medical school and starting a career in medicine?

I love those people. They're young, they're enthusiastic, they're committed. But a funny thing is happening. The vast majority are taking salaried positions in medical groups rather than starting their own practices. I used to do salaried medicine and my experience was that it doesn't give you the freedom to practice the way you want. (I still did it my way back then, but I got flack for it constantly.) So I would say to these young doctors, "You have made a wonderful decision to become a doctor, and the real joy and satisfaction of that profession will be in the care and commitment you have toward your patients and toward the people you come in contact with. If you want to really be happy and joyful as a doctor, do it in a way that does not compromise the quality of care that you provide. Be the best doctor you can be and I think the rest will come naturally."

And if you could bring a message to current physicians in the U.S., what would it be?

My message to physicians would be that this is a very honorable, wonderful profession. You have chosen a profession in which you can help people all day long, every day of your life. You are in a position to really advise people and do things for people that will enhance their lives. You can take away pain, you can cure illness, you can help people understand their health, you can work with their mental health. You have been given tremendous gifts, and to respect that and not compromise that and to really be the best doctor you can be requires that you open your heart and feel compassion, love and kindness for your patient. If you do that, I think all the success you want will be there as well. It will be automatic.